The Sourdough Discard Cookbook

Easy Recipes to Use Your Starter Discard for Pancakes, Muffins, Crackers and Everyday Baking

by LeeAnn Baker

Medialusion Books

COPYRIGHT

TABLE OF CONTENTS

Introduction

IT IS AN INGREDIENT. A GOOD ONE.

If you keep a sourdough starter, even a neglected, occasionally forgotten, sometimes crusty one, you produce discard constantly. Every time you feed your starter, you remove a portion to keep the colony manageable and the yeast healthy. That removed portion is your discard. It still contains wild yeast. It still contains lactic acid bacteria. It still has flavor, acidity, and a complex microbial character that commercial yeast simply cannot replicate. The only thing it doesn't have, in meaningful quantity, is the leavening power of a freshly fed, fully active starter.

That distinction matters. It is the whole reason this book exists.

Because once you understand what discard actually is, and what it can and cannot do, every recipe in this book makes immediate, logical sense. You stop guessing. You stop wondering why the pancakes came out dense or why the crackers softened overnight. You understand the material you're working with, and that understanding turns a frustrating guessing game into something genuinely fun.

> *This book is not about making do with leftovers. It is about using a remarkable ingredient on purpose.*

The recipes you'll find here were chosen because they play to discard's actual strengths: its tang, its tenderness, its ability to add complexity to baked goods without announcing itself. Every recipe in this book is designed to be made with cold discard, straight from the refrigerator, without any pre-warming, activation, or planning ahead. You can decide at 7 a.m. that you want pancakes and have them on the table by 7:30. You can pull crackers together on a Tuesday afternoon before a last-minute gathering. The fridge is always your starting point.

What you will not find here are recipes that require you to coddle your discard, wait for it to "wake up," or worry about whether it's active enough. That's starter territory. Discard is more relaxed than that, and once you start cooking with it that way, you will be too.

HOW THIS BOOK IS ORGANIZED

The book opens with two short foundation chapters before any recipes appear. Chapter 1 covers what you actually need to know about discard, storage, lifespan, the difference between discard and active starter, and how to build up enough of it for larger batches. Chapter 2 teaches you to read your specific discard: how thick or thin it is, how sour, and how to adjust any recipe in the book to match what you have on hand today.

These chapters are short on purpose. They cover only what is genuinely useful before you start baking, and nothing more.

The recipe chapters are organized by category rather than by occasion, because discard doesn't care about occasion. Breakfast comes first because it represents the fastest, most reliable discard wins, dishes that go from refrigerator to table in under forty minutes with minimal effort. Crackers and flatbreads come next because they are the most forgiving category in the book: tolerant of a wide range of discard ages, hydration levels, and sourness, and almost impossible to completely ruin. Sweet bakes and desserts follow, then a smaller chapter of savory bites, and finally a chapter of master formulas, three core batters with variation tables that effectively multiply your recipe options without requiring you to learn entirely new techniques.

The book closes with Chapter 8: the Troubleshooting Master Guide. If a recipe doesn't turn out the way you expected, that chapter is where you go. It is organized by symptom, not by recipe, not by chapter, so you can find your specific problem quickly and understand both the fix and the reason it happened in the first place. No other sourdough discard book currently in print offers this kind of systematic troubleshooting support. We built it because the reader research was unambiguous: when recipes fail and there's nowhere to turn, people don't try again. We want you to try again.

WHAT YOU NEED BEFORE YOU START

The equipment list for this book is intentionally short. You do not need a stand mixer, a proofing drawer, a kitchen scale calibrated to the gram, or any piece of equipment that doesn't already live in a well-stocked home kitchen. These are the things that will genuinely make a difference:

- A digital kitchen scale. Baking is chemistry, and volume measurements, cups and tablespoons, are imprecise in ways that matter in baked goods. Every recipe in this book provides both weight and volume measurements, but weight is always more accurate. A basic digital scale costs less than fifteen dollars and will improve every recipe you make, in this book and outside it.
- A standard set of dry and liquid measuring cups and spoons, for the moments when you don't want to use the scale.
- Two mixing bowls, one large, one medium.
- A rubber spatula and a whisk.
- A cast iron skillet or heavy-bottomed pan for stovetop recipes.
- A standard rimmed half-sheet pan (18 x 13 inches) for crackers and sheet-pan recipes.
- A 9 x 5-inch loaf pan and a standard 12-cup muffin tin for the quick bread and muffin recipes.
- Parchment paper. Non-negotiable for crackers. Highly recommended for everything else.

That is the complete list. If you have all of those things, you can make every recipe in this book without buying a single additional tool.

For ingredients, the same principle applies. Every recipe was written around pantry staples available at any grocery store: all-purpose flour, butter, eggs, sugar, salt, baking soda, baking powder, and a handful of common spices and flavorings. Where a recipe calls for something slightly less common, rye flour, for example, or a specific type of cheese, it always includes a substitution note. Nothing in these pages requires a specialty store or an online order.

A NOTE ON SOURNESS

One of the most consistent complaints in reviews of sourdough discard cookbooks, and I read hundreds of them while developing this one, is that the recipes taste too sour. The tang overwhelms the other flavors. The discard makes its presence known in a way that isn't pleasant.

This is almost always a discard age problem, not a recipe problem.

Discard gets more acidic the longer it sits. A one-day-old discard has a mild, yogurt-like tang. A ten-day-old discard has a sharp, almost vinegary bite. Both are perfectly usable, but not interchangeably. The older discard belongs in recipes that can handle its intensity: crackers with bold toppings, chocolate cake where the bitterness reads as depth, rye flatbreads where the tang is part of the flavor profile. The younger discard belongs in recipes where you want the discard's character to be subtle: delicate muffins, shortbread, crepes.

Chapter 2 walks you through this in detail. The appendix at the back of the book includes an index that organizes every recipe by the discard age it works best with, so you can always match what you have to what you should make today.

The short version: if something tasted too sour, use younger discard next time. If something tasted flat and you wanted more complexity, reach for the older jar. Once you have that one variable under control, the sourness issue disappears entirely.

The discard is not the problem. The mismatch between the discard and the recipe is the problem. This book is designed to eliminate that mismatch.

✦ ✦ ✦

HOW TO USE THIS BOOK

If you are new to baking with sourdough discard, start with Chapters 1 and 2. They are short, you can read both in twenty minutes, and they will make every recipe you attempt afterward more successful. Then go to Chapter 3 and make the Classic Sourdough Discard Pancakes. They are the fastest possible demonstration of what discard can do, and they are nearly impossible to get wrong.

If you are an experienced sourdough baker who already understands your starter and your discard, feel free to skip directly to the recipe chapters. Skim Chapter 2 for the Quick Discard Assessment checklist, it's a useful sixty-second habit to build before any bake, and then cook whatever looks good.

If a recipe doesn't work out, go to Chapter 8. Find your symptom. Read the diagnosis. Try again.

That's the whole system. It is not complicated, because it doesn't need to be. The ingredient you're working with, that jar you've been pushing to the back of the fridge, is more capable than you've been giving it credit for.

- Let's put it to work.

CHAPTER 1

Discard Foundations

Before we get to recipes, there are a few things worth understanding about the ingredient you're working with. This chapter covers what sourdough discard actually is, how it differs from active starter, how long you can keep it and how to store it properly, and how to accumulate enough of it for the recipes in this book. None of this is complicated. Read it once, and you'll have everything you need.

WHAT SOURDOUGH DISCARD ACTUALLY IS

A sourdough starter is a living culture of wild yeast and lactic acid bacteria suspended in a mixture of flour and water. To keep that culture healthy and active, you feed it regularly, typically by discarding a portion of the existing starter and adding fresh flour and water. The portion you remove is your discard.

Here is what discard still contains when you take it out of the jar:

- Wild yeast, though in lower concentration than in a freshly fed, active starter
- Lactic acid bacteria, which produce the lactic and acetic acids responsible for sourdough's characteristic tang
- Partially fermented flour with broken-down gluten structures that contribute to tender, soft textures in baked goods
- Complex organic acids that act as natural flavor enhancers and mild preservatives

Here is what discard does not have in useful quantity:

- Sufficient leavening power to raise a bread loaf on its own, the yeast population has declined since the last feeding and is not vigorous enough to generate the gas production a proper loaf requires

That single limitation defines what discard is good for and what it isn't. It is not a substitute for active starter in yeasted bread recipes. It is an exceptional ingredient for pancakes, muffins, crackers, cakes, cookies, and flatbreads, anything that uses chemical leaveners like baking soda or baking powder to rise, or anything that doesn't need to rise at all.

> *Think of discard as a flavor ingredient first, and a structural ingredient second. It makes things taste better, and it makes their texture more interesting. What it does not do is lift a loaf of bread.*

DISCARD VS. ACTIVE STARTER: THE PRACTICAL DIFFERENCE

The distinction between discard and active starter confuses a lot of bakers, and competing books rarely explain it clearly. Here is the practical version:

Active starter has been recently fed, usually within the past four to eight hours, and is at or near its peak of fermentation activity. It is bubbly, slightly domed on top, and has roughly doubled in volume since its last feeding. This is the starter you use for traditional sourdough bread, where fermentation-driven leavening is the entire point.

Sourdough discard is everything else: starter that hasn't been recently fed, starter removed during a feeding, or starter that has been sitting in the refrigerator for anywhere from a few hours to a couple of weeks. It may have some bubble activity, or none at all. It has not peaked. It will not reliably leaven a loaf of bread. But it has something active starter doesn't always have in abundance: concentrated flavor.

The longer discard sits before you use it, the more acidic and tangy it becomes. Fresh discard, used the same day it was removed from the starter jar, has a mild, yogurt-like sourness. Week-old refrigerator discard has a sharper, more pronounced tang. Both are useful. The question is which recipe they belong in, and Chapter 2 covers exactly that.

Can You Use Active Starter in These Recipes?

Yes. Any recipe in this book that calls for sourdough discard will also work with active starter. The flavor may be slightly less complex, and in sweet recipes you may notice slightly less tang, which is usually a good thing. The one situation where it matters: if your active starter is very recently fed and extremely bubbly, add it to the recipe immediately rather than letting it sit, to avoid it over-fermenting before you bake.

STORING YOUR DISCARD

Refrigerator Storage

The refrigerator is your primary discard storage environment, and it's more forgiving than most people realize. Cold temperatures slow the fermentation process dramatically, which means discard sitting in a refrigerator jar is changing, but slowly. A properly stored discard can remain usable for up to two weeks.

The container matters more than most people think. Discard stored in a loosely covered bowl or a container that isn't airtight will dry out on the surface, form a thick skin, and pick up refrigerator odors. Use a jar with a lid, mason jars are ideal, and leave an inch or two of headspace at the top. The discard will continue producing small amounts of gas even in the refrigerator, and a fully sealed container with no headspace can build pressure.

Stir the discard before you use it. A layer of liquid, greyish or slightly translucent, often separates and rises to the top after a few days. This liquid is called hooch, and it is simply alcohol produced by the yeast during slow fermentation. It is not a sign that the discard has gone bad. Stir it back in and proceed. If the discard underneath smells sharply of vinegar with no sour-dairy undertone, it's very old but still usually usable in strongly flavored recipes. If it smells rotten, not tangy, not vinegary, but genuinely foul, or if you see pink, orange, or red streaks in it, discard the discard. That coloring indicates bacterial contamination that has nothing to do with healthy fermentation.

Freezer Storage

Freezing discard is an underused strategy that solves one of the most common discard problems: you have more than you can use, or you're going to be away for a few weeks and don't want to lose what you've accumulated.

Discard freezes well for up to three months with no meaningful loss of quality. The lactic acid bacteria go dormant in the freezer and reactivate when thawed. The flavor profile is preserved. Frozen-and-thawed discard performs identically to fresh refrigerator discard in every recipe in this book.

To freeze discard: pour it into a zip-lock freezer bag in measured portions, half-cup or one-cup amounts work well, press out the air, label with the date, and lay flat in the freezer. Flat frozen discard stacks efficiently and thaws quickly. To thaw, move the bag to the refrigerator the night before you plan to bake, or set it in a bowl of cool water for thirty to forty-five minutes if you need it faster. Do not microwave to thaw, the heat will kill the yeast and bacteria and flatten the flavor.

Accumulating Enough Discard

Most recipes in this book call for between half a cup and one cup (120–240 grams) of discard. If you feed your starter once a day and discard roughly half each time, you're generating about a cup of discard per feeding. One week of daily feedings gives you more than enough for a full baking session.

If you don't bake frequently enough to use discard as fast as you produce it: freeze it in batches. When you're ready for a big baking day, thaw what you need. This is the most efficient approach for intermittent bakers, and it means you never have to throw discard away.

Use the reference chart below to match your storage situation to the right approach:

Storage Method	Container	Usable Lifespan	Signs It's Gone	Best For
Refrigerator	Airtight jar or container	**Up to** 2 weeks	Pink/orange streaks, foul smell (not just sour)	Everyday baking
Freezer	Zip-lock bag or freezer container	**Up to** 3 months	Freezer burn, off smell after thawing	Large-batch recipes, long gaps between baking
Room temperature	Any covered bowl	**Up to** 8 hours	Bubbles aggressively then collapses, use it now	Baking same day only

UNDERSTANDING YOUR FEEDING SCHEDULE

How often you feed your starter determines how much discard you generate and how old that discard is by the time you use it. There is no universal correct feeding schedule, it depends on where you keep your starter, how often you bake, and how much maintenance time you want to invest.

Room-Temperature Starters

A starter kept at room temperature needs feeding every twelve to twenty-four hours to stay healthy and active. This produces more discard more frequently, ideal if you bake often, challenging if you don't. Room-temperature discard that you're not using immediately should go into the refrigerator within a few hours. Left out, it will ferment quickly and become very sour, then eventually become too acidic even for the bacteria to survive in.

Refrigerator Starters

Most home bakers who don't bake bread every day keep their starter in the refrigerator between uses, feeding it once a week or even less frequently. Refrigerator starters produce less frequent discard but often produce discard with more developed, complex flavor because the slow cold fermentation allows acid development over a longer period. This is the most common setup for the recipes in this book, pull the starter out of the fridge, feed it, remove the discard, and either use the discard immediately or store it back in the refrigerator.

The Zero-Waste Weekly Rhythm

Here is a simple framework that works for most home bakers using this book:

- Feed your starter once a week, on whatever day works for your schedule.
- When you feed, remove your discard into a dedicated discard jar in the refrigerator rather than throwing it away.
- Once a week, or whenever the discard jar gets full, bake something from this book.
- If the jar gets ahead of you, freeze what you have and start fresh.

This rhythm produces enough discard for one solid baking session per week, generates essentially zero waste, and requires no more planning than you're probably already doing for your starter.

You don't need to bake on a schedule. You need a system that turns your existing starter routine into usable ingredients automatically. The discard jar in the refrigerator is that system.

A NOTE ON FLOUR

The flour you use to feed your starter, and therefore the flour composition of your discard, affects how it behaves in recipes. Most home bakers feed with all-purpose flour, which is what the recipes in this book are calibrated to. If you feed your starter with whole wheat, rye, or a mix, your discard will be slightly denser, slightly more flavorful, and slightly more acidic than all-purpose-fed discard.

None of this is a problem. The differences are noticeable but not dramatic, and the troubleshooting guide in Chapter 8 covers specific adjustments if you find your whole-grain-fed discard is consistently producing baked goods that are denser or more sour than you'd like. As a general rule: whole-grain-fed discard is excellent in crackers, flatbreads, and strongly flavored baked goods. For delicate recipes like crepes or shortbread, all-purpose-fed discard produces a more neutral, predictable result.

WHAT YOU NOW KNOW

Discard is a living ingredient with flavor, acidity, and tenderizing properties, but not enough leavening power to raise a loaf of bread on its own. It stores well in the refrigerator for up to two weeks, freezes for up to three months, and accumulates naturally from any regular feeding routine. The older it gets, the more sour it becomes, which matters for recipe selection. And the flour you feed your starter with influences the character of your discard in ways that are useful to understand but easy to work around.

That's everything you need from this chapter. Chapter 2 takes the next step: teaching you to look at your specific discard, today, in your jar, and understand exactly what you have before you start baking.

CHAPTER 2

Reading Your Discard

Every jar of sourdough discard is different. Yours is influenced by the flour you use, the temperature of your kitchen, how long it's been sitting in the refrigerator, and the particular wild yeast and bacteria that colonized your starter over time. No two discard jars are identical, which means a recipe that works perfectly with one baker's week-old discard might turn out denser or more sour in the hands of another baker using discard from a different jar.

This is not a flaw in sourdough baking. It is the nature of working with a living ingredient. And it is entirely manageable once you know what to look for.

This chapter teaches you to assess your discard before you start baking, not with a pH meter or a laboratory instrument, but with your eyes, your nose, and a spoon. The assessment takes sixty seconds and answers three questions. Those three answers tell you which recipes your discard is best suited for today, and what adjustments to make if you want to use it in something outside its ideal range.

QUESTION ONE: HOW THICK IS IT?

Hydration is the ratio of water to flour in your discard, and it varies significantly depending on how you maintain your starter. A starter fed with equal weights of flour and water (called 100% hydration) produces discard that pours like a thick pancake batter. A stiffer starter fed with more flour than water produces discard closer to the consistency of peanut butter. A looser, high-hydration starter produces discard that pours almost like cream.

The recipes in this book are calibrated for 100% hydration discard, the most common home baker setup. If your discard is significantly thicker or thinner than a pourable pancake batter, small adjustments keep everything on track.

If Your Discard Is Very Thick

Thick discard, the kind that holds its shape when dropped from a spoon, contains more flour relative to water than the recipes expect. Left unadjusted, it can make baked goods slightly denser and drier than intended. The fix is simple: thin it with water before measuring. Add water one tablespoon at a time, stirring between additions, until the discard reaches a consistency closer to thick pancake batter. Then measure the amount the recipe calls for.

Alternatively, and this is often easier, reduce the flour in the recipe by one to two tablespoons per cup of discard you're using. The effect is the same: you're rebalancing the ratio of wet to dry ingredients.

If Your Discard Is Very Thin

Thin discard, watery, almost pourable, barely thicker than milk, contains less flour relative to water. Left unadjusted, it can make baked goods slightly wetter or cause them to spread more than intended, particularly in cookie and cracker recipes. Two options: either stir a tablespoon of flour into the discard before measuring, or reduce the liquid the recipe calls for by a tablespoon or two.

For most recipes, especially pancakes, muffins, and cakes, thinner discard makes very little practical difference and requires no adjustment at all. It matters most in crackers (where excess moisture prevents crisping) and cookies (where it can cause spreading).

The Spoon Test

Not sure how to classify your discard's thickness? Use the spoon test: dip a spoon into your discard and lift it out. If the discard falls off in one continuous ribbon that holds its shape for a moment before settling, that's the target consistency, roughly 100% hydration. If it runs off immediately like water, it's thin. If it falls in a single slow blob and piles up in the jar, it's thick.

QUESTION TWO: HOW SOUR IS IT?

Sourness is the variable that causes the most recipe failures in sourdough discard baking, not because sour discard is bad, but because bakers use it in recipes where the tang has nowhere to hide and no counterbalance to soften it.

Understanding your discard's sourness level takes literally five seconds: open the jar, smell it, and taste a small amount off the tip of a spoon. You are placing it in one of three categories.

Mild — smells like yogurt or cultured buttermilk, with a gentle, clean tang. Tastes slightly creamy and sour without sharpness. This is fresh discard: one to three days out of the refrigerator, or discard from a starter that is fed frequently and kept cold. Mild discard is versatile, it works in everything from delicate shortbread to bold crackers, because its sourness won't overwhelm any flavor profile.

Medium — smells tangy and sharp, noticeably more acidic than yogurt. Tastes clearly sour with some complexity underneath. This is most home bakers' everyday discard: four to seven days old, produced by a weekly-fed refrigerator starter. It is the sweet spot for most recipes in this book, enough flavor to be interesting, not so much that it dominates.

Tangy — smells assertively sour, almost vinegary. Has a sharp, pronounced bite. This is older discard: seven to fourteen days in the refrigerator, or discard from a warmer environment that ferments faster. Tangy discard is not a problem. It is an asset in the right recipes, crackers, rye flatbreads, pretzels, chocolate cake. In delicate recipes, it will overwhelm.

The table below maps each sourness profile to the recipes it works best in:

Profile	Age	Smell	Taste	Best Recipes
Mild	1–3 days	Yogurt-like, light tang	Gently sour, slightly creamy	Crepes, shortbread, muffins, pancakes, cakes
Medium	4–7 days	Tangy, pleasantly sharp	Noticeably sour, complex	Waffles, cookies, flatbreads, pizza dough, scones
Tangy	7–14 days	Sharp, almost vinegary	Assertively sour, bold	Crackers, rye flatbreads, chocolate cake, pretzels

You don't need to change your discard to match a recipe. You need to match your recipe to your discard. The appendix at the back of this book indexes every recipe by the discard profile it works best with, use it.

QUESTION THREE: DOES IT SMELL RIGHT?

The third assessment is the most important one, and also the fastest. Before you use any discard, smell it.

Healthy discard, regardless of age, smells like some variation of the following: sour, tangy, yeasty, slightly alcoholic, reminiscent of beer or vinegar or yogurt. These are all normal. What you are listening for, with your nose, is any smell that falls outside this spectrum.

Discard that has gone bad does not smell sour. It smells wrong in a way that is hard to describe but instantly recognizable, foul, putrid, musty, or chemical in a way that has nothing to do with fermentation. If you encounter this smell, do not use the discard. Throw it out, wash the jar thoroughly, and start your discard jar fresh with the next feeding.

The visual check goes alongside the smell test: if you see pink, orange, red, or black spots or streaks in your discard, not the grey-brown surface liquid that is normal hooch, but actual colored growth, that is contamination. It is rare in a healthy sourdough routine, but it does happen occasionally, particularly if the jar wasn't clean when you started or if something else got into the discard. Again: throw it out.

A thin layer of grey or slightly brownish liquid on the surface of refrigerator discard is hooch, alcohol produced during slow fermentation. It is completely normal, harmless, and easy to deal with. Stir it back in before measuring. If it's present in large amounts, your discard is older and likely in the "tangy" category.

THE QUICK DISCARD ASSESSMENT

Run through these three questions before every bake. Takes 60 seconds.

1. How thick is my discard?

□ Very thick (holds its shape) → thin with water, or reduce flour in recipe by 1–2 tbsp

□ Pancake batter consistency → no adjustment needed

□ Very thin (watery) → add 1 tbsp flour to discard, or reduce recipe liquid by 1–2 tbsp

2. How sour is my discard?

□ Mild (yogurt-like) → any recipe in the book; ideal for delicate bakes

□ Medium (tangy, sharp) → most recipes; the everyday sweet spot

□ Tangy (assertively sour) → crackers, flatbreads, chocolate cake, pretzels; avoid delicate recipes

3. Does it smell right?

□ Smells sour, tangy, yeasty, or slightly alcoholic → good to go

□ Has a grey liquid layer on top → normal hooch; stir in and proceed

□ Smells foul, putrid, or chemical → discard it. Do not use.

MAKING ADJUSTMENTS IN REAL TIME

The assessment above tells you what you have. Sometimes what you have isn't quite ideal for the recipe you want to make. Here is how to close that gap without abandoning the recipe or waiting until you have different discard.

Dialing Down Sourness

If your discard is tangier than ideal for a particular recipe, you have several options depending on the recipe type:

- **Add fat.** Butter, oil, or cream coat the palate and suppress the perception of acidity. Recipes with higher fat content naturally mask sourness better. Adding an extra tablespoon of butter to a muffin batter can meaningfully soften an assertive discard.
- **Add sugar.** Sweetness counterbalances acidity. In recipes that already call for sugar, you can increase it slightly, by a tablespoon or two, to soften tangy discard without changing the texture of the bake.
- **Reduce the discard.** If a recipe calls for one cup and your discard is very tangy, use three-quarters of a cup and make up the difference with an equal weight of plain flour and water mixed together. You preserve the discard's flavor contribution while diluting its intensity.

- **Choose a different recipe.** The appendix indexes every recipe by discard profile. If your discard is very tangy, let that guide your recipe choice rather than fighting the ingredient.

Dialing Up Sourness

If your discard is milder than you'd like, particularly for recipes where you want a more pronounced sourdough character, these approaches add complexity:

- **Use older discard.** If your current discard is fresh and mild, let it sit in the refrigerator for another two or three days before using it. The additional fermentation time increases acidity naturally.

- **Add a small amount of rye flour.** Rye ferments faster and more aggressively than all-purpose flour, contributing additional lactic acid character. Swapping one or two tablespoons of the recipe's flour for dark rye flour adds noticeable complexity, particularly in crackers and flatbreads.

- **Extend the batter's rest time.** For pancakes, waffles, or flatbread doughs, mixing the batter and letting it rest at room temperature for thirty to sixty minutes before cooking allows additional fermentation and deepens the flavor. Cover the bowl and let it sit, you'll notice the difference.

YOU'RE READY TO BAKE

That is the complete assessment system. Three questions, sixty seconds, and you know exactly what your discard needs and which recipes will work best with it today. Run through the Quick Discard Assessment before every bake, not because something will necessarily go wrong if you skip it, but because it builds the intuition that eventually makes you a confident, adaptive baker rather than someone who follows recipes rigidly and panics when results vary.

The recipes begin in the next chapter. Breakfast first, because it's where most people start, because the recipes are fast, and because there is almost nothing more satisfying than sourdough discard pancakes on a Saturday morning when you weren't expecting to make anything at all.

CHAPTER 3

Breakfast First

Breakfast is where most people first discover what sourdough discard can do, and why it's worth keeping.

The recipes in this chapter are designed around one constraint: your discard comes straight from the refrigerator. No pre-warming, no activation, no waiting for anything to come to room temperature. You open the jar, measure what you need, and start mixing. From refrigerator to table, most of these recipes take thirty to forty minutes. The rest take under an hour.

That matters because the main reason people throw discard away isn't that they don't want to use it. It's that using it feels like it requires planning they didn't do. These recipes remove that obstacle entirely. The discard is ready when you are, not the other way around.

The chapter moves through four categories: pancakes and waffles, which are the fastest and most reliable discard recipes in existence; muffins and quick breads, which take slightly longer but reward you with something that keeps well for days; breakfast savories, for the mornings when sweet isn't what you want; and biscuits, which occupy their own category because they are simultaneously one of the simplest and most satisfying things you can make with discard.

The best thing about sourdough discard pancakes is that they don't taste like a compromise. They taste like the actual reason people keep starters in the first place.

A note on the recipes that follow: each one includes both weight (grams) and volume (cups and tablespoons) measurements. Use weight whenever you can, the results are more consistent. But volume measurements are here for the moments when the scale isn't on the counter and you're not going to go get it.

PANCAKES & WAFFLES

01 CLASSIC SOURDOUGH DISCARD PANCAKES

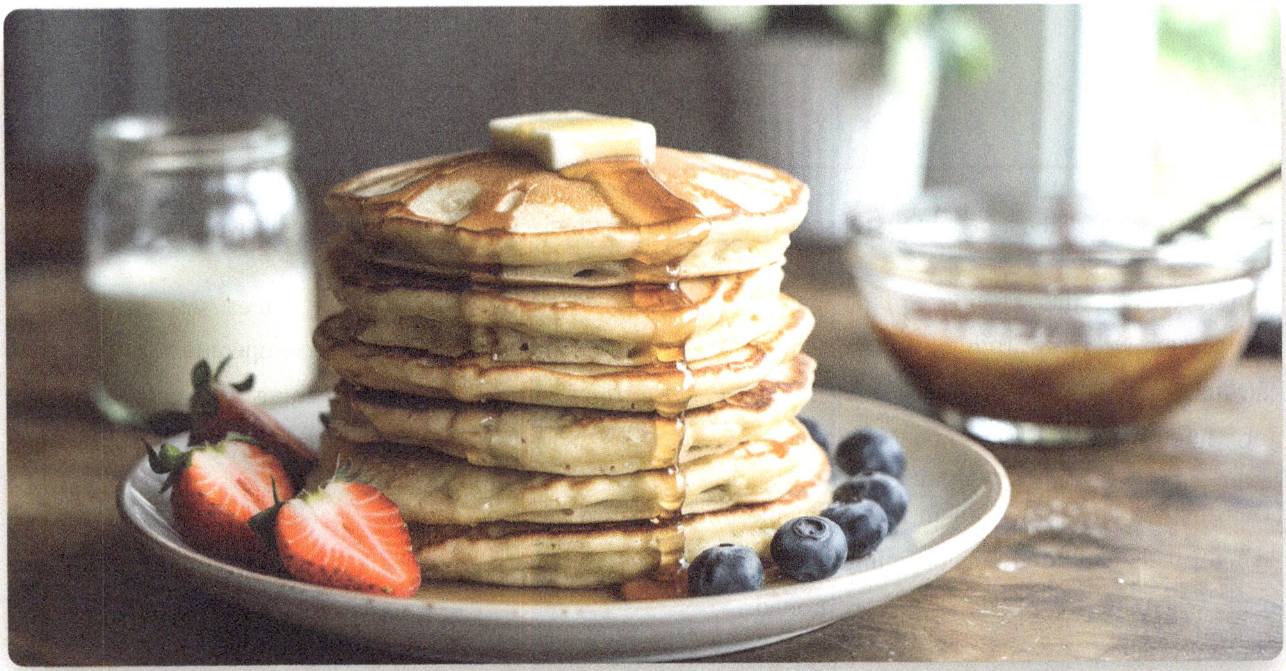

This is the recipe to start with. It is reliable, fast, and produces pancakes with a subtle tang and a texture that commercial mixes cannot replicate, slightly crispy at the edges, tender in the center, and just sour enough to be interesting. Master this one first. The five variations that follow it are built on the same foundation.

PREP TIME	COOK TIME	YIELD	DISCARD
10 minutes	20 minutes	10–12 pancakes	Mild to medium

INGREDIENTS

1 cup (240 g) sourdough discard, cold from the refrigerator
1 cup (120 g) all-purpose flour
1 tablespoon (12 g) granulated sugar
1 teaspoon (5 g) baking powder
½ teaspoon (3 g) baking soda

½ teaspoon (3 g) fine salt
1 large egg
¾ cup (180 ml) whole milk
2 tablespoons (28 g) unsalted butter, melted and cooled slightly
1 teaspoon (5 ml) pure vanilla extract

INSTRUCTIONS

1. In a large bowl, whisk together the flour, sugar, baking powder, baking soda, and salt. Set aside.

2. In a separate medium bowl or large measuring cup, whisk together the sourdough discard, egg, milk, melted butter, and vanilla extract until smooth and fully combined.

3. Pour the wet ingredients into the dry ingredients and stir with a spatula until just combined. Stop as soon as the dry flour disappears, the batter will be lumpy, and that is exactly right. Overmixed pancake batter produces flat, tough pancakes. A few streaks of flour are fine; they will hydrate as the batter rests.

4. Let the batter rest for five minutes while you heat your pan. Place a large skillet or griddle over medium heat and add a small amount of butter or neutral oil. The pan is ready when a drop of water flicked onto the surface bounces and evaporates immediately.

5. Pour approximately ¼ cup of batter per pancake onto the hot surface. Cook until bubbles form across the surface of the pancake and the edges look set, about two to three minutes. Flip once and cook for another one to two minutes, until the underside is golden brown.

6. Serve immediately, or keep warm in a 200°F (95°C) oven on a sheet pan while you finish the batch.

BAKER'S TIP

If your first pancake comes out pale and flat, your pan isn't hot enough. If it comes out dark brown in under a minute, reduce the heat slightly. The first pancake is always a calibration pancake, eat it in the kitchen and adjust before you serve the rest.

Storage: Cooked pancakes keep in the refrigerator for up to 3 days. Reheat in a toaster or a 325°F oven for 5 minutes. They also freeze beautifully: cool completely, stack with parchment between each pancake, seal in a zip-lock bag, and freeze for up to 2 months. Reheat from frozen in the toaster.

Nutritional Information (per pancake, based on 12 pancakes)

Calories	Protein	Carbs	Fat	Fiber	Sodium
185	6 g	27 g	6 g	1 g	290 mg

VARIATIONS ON THE CLASSIC PANCAKE

Each variation below uses the Classic Sourdough Discard Pancake recipe as its base. Only the changes from that recipe are listed.

02 BLUEBERRY LEMON RICOTTA PANCAKES

Ricotta makes these substantially thicker and richer than the classic. The lemon zest cuts through the discard's tang in a way that makes the whole thing taste deliberately bright rather than accidentally sour.

PREP TIME	COOK TIME	YIELD	DISCARD
12 minutes	25 minutes	8–10 pancakes	Mild

Changes from Classic Recipe

- Replace the milk with ½ cup (120 g) whole-milk ricotta + ½ cup (120 ml) whole milk, whisked together until smooth
- Add the zest of 1 large lemon to the wet ingredients
- Fold 1 cup (150 g) fresh or frozen blueberries into the finished batter (do not thaw frozen berries first, they will bleed into the batter and turn it grey)
- Reduce vanilla to ½ teaspoon

METHOD NOTES

1. The batter will be noticeably thicker than the classic version. Use a slightly lower heat setting, medium-low rather than medium, and allow a full three to four minutes per side. The ricotta needs time to set. These pancakes are thicker and more fragile when raw; flip them carefully.
2. Storage: Refrigerate up to 2 days. Freeze up to 2 months as described in Recipe 01.

Nutritional Information (per pancake, based on 9 pancakes)

Calories	Protein	Carbs	Fat	Fiber	Sodium
210	8 g	28 g	7 g	1 g	270 mg

03 SAVORY SCALLION & CHEDDAR PANCAKES

These are not breakfast-sweet pancakes with a savory ingredient thrown in. They are genuinely savory, closer to a Korean pajeon than to a diner short stack, and they work as breakfast, lunch, or a side dish alongside soup or eggs.

PREP TIME 10 minutes	COOK TIME 20 minutes	YIELD 8–10 pancakes	DISCARD Medium

Changes from Classic Recipe

- Omit the sugar and vanilla
- Reduce milk to ½ cup (120 ml)
- Add ½ teaspoon (1 g) freshly ground black pepper and ¼ teaspoon (0.5 g) garlic powder to the dry ingredients
- Fold into the finished batter: 4 scallions, thinly sliced (about ½ cup / 50 g); ¾ cup (85 g) shredded sharp cheddar
- Use neutral oil (not butter) for the pan

METHOD NOTES

1. Cook over medium heat the same way as the classic. These pancakes will not bubble across the surface the way sweet pancakes do, watch the edges instead. When the edges look dry and the underside lifts cleanly from the pan, it's time to flip. Serve with sour cream or hot sauce.
2. Storage: Refrigerate up to 3 days. Reheat in a skillet over medium heat rather than the toaster, they re-crisp better that way. Do not freeze; the cheese texture suffers.

Nutritional Information (per pancake, based on 9 pancakes)

Calories	Protein	Carbs	Fat	Fiber	Sodium
195	8 g	22 g	8 g	1 g	380 mg

04 CRISPY BELGIAN-STYLE WAFFLES

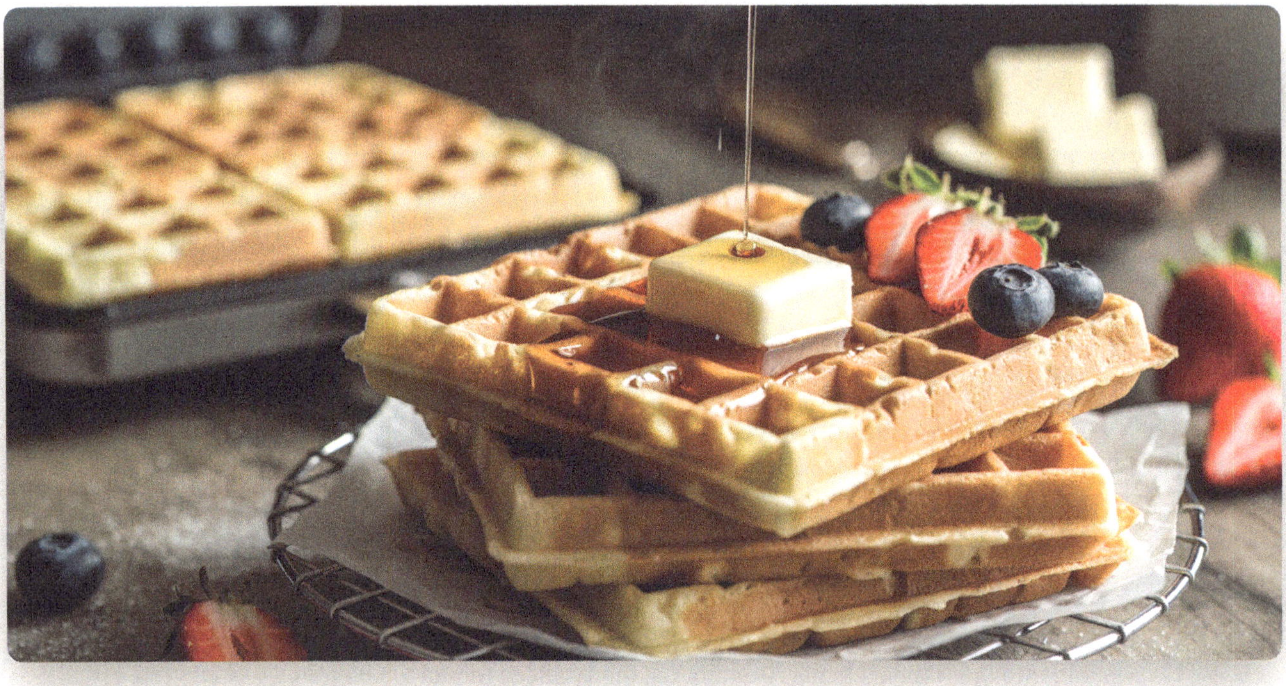

The sourdough discard does two things in this recipe that commercial waffle mix cannot: it adds flavor complexity, and its acidity reacts with the baking soda to produce an especially vigorous rise inside the waffle iron, which means a genuinely crispy exterior and a light, airy interior. Do not stack these waffles, they steam each other and go soft immediately.

PREP TIME	COOK TIME	YIELD	DISCARD
10 minutes	25 minutes	6 waffles	Mild to medium

INGREDIENTS

1 cup (240 g) sourdough discard, cold
1½ cups (180 g) all-purpose flour
2 tablespoons (24 g) granulated sugar
1½ teaspoons (7 g) baking powder
½ teaspoon (3 g) baking soda
½ teaspoon (3 g) fine salt
2 large eggs, separated
¾ cup (180 ml) whole milk

6 tablespoons (85 g) unsalted butter, melted
1 teaspoon (5 ml) pure vanilla extract

INSTRUCTIONS

1. Preheat your waffle iron according to its instructions. Whisk together the flour, sugar, baking powder, baking soda, and salt in a large bowl.
2. In a separate bowl, whisk together the egg yolks, discard, milk, melted butter, and vanilla until smooth.
3. In a third bowl, clean and grease-free, beat the egg whites with a hand mixer or whisk until they hold soft peaks. This step is what makes Belgian waffles genuinely light rather than dense. Do not skip it.
4. Pour the wet ingredients into the dry and stir until just combined. Fold in the egg whites in two additions, using a spatula and a gentle hand. Some white streaks are fine.
5. Grease the waffle iron lightly with butter or cooking spray. Pour the batter in according to your iron's capacity, usually about ¾ cup per waffle. Close the lid and cook until the steam from the iron slows significantly and the waffle lifts cleanly without resistance, about 4–5 minutes depending on your iron.
6. Transfer immediately to a wire rack, not a plate, while you cook the remaining waffles.

BAKER'S TIP

If your waffles are sticking: the iron isn't hot enough, or you're opening it too early. Wait until the steaming stops almost completely before checking. If waffles are consistently sticking despite good timing, increase the butter in the batter by one tablespoon.

Storage: Cool completely on a rack before storing. Refrigerate up to 3 days or freeze up to 3 months. Reheat from frozen directly in the toaster, this is actually the best way to re-crisp them.

Nutritional Information (per waffle)

Calories	Protein	Carbs	Fat	Fiber	Sodium
295	8 g	36 g	13 g	1 g	340 mg

05 OVERNIGHT OAT WAFFLES

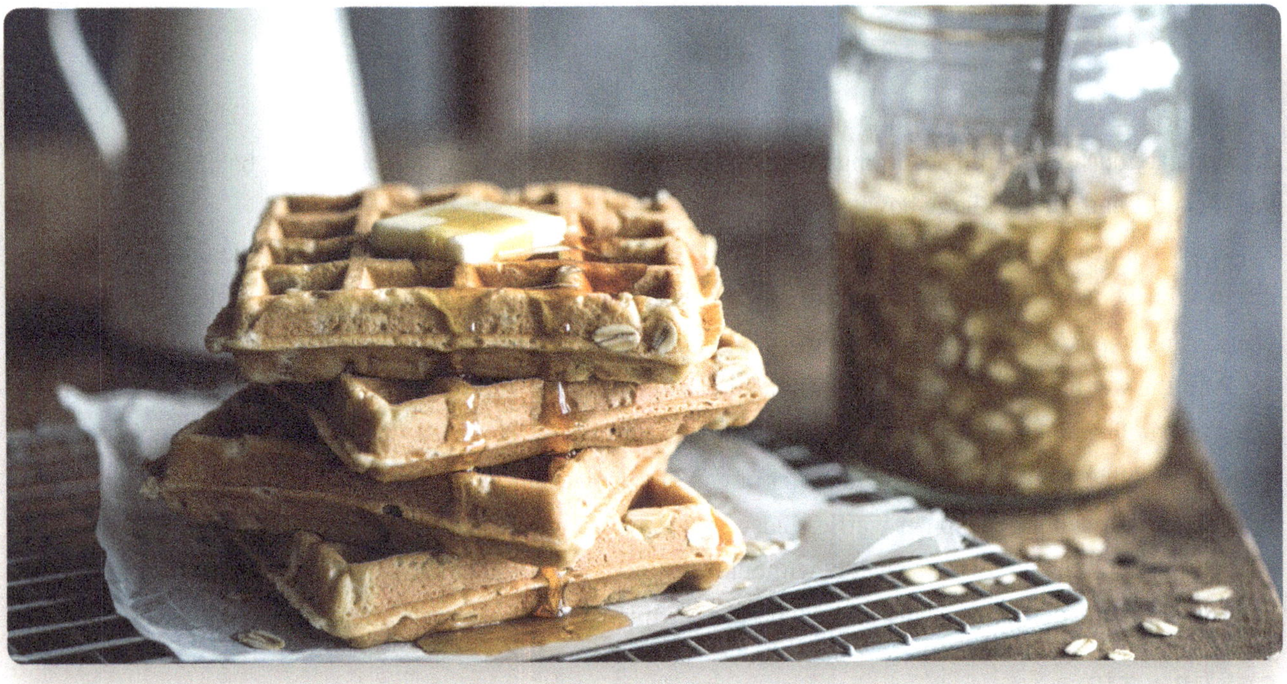

This is the one recipe in the breakfast chapter that requires a small amount of advance planning, you mix the oat base the night before. In exchange, you get waffles in the morning with almost no active effort, and a texture that is substantially heartier and more complex than a standard waffle. The oats soften overnight in the discard and create a batter with more chew and more staying power than all-flour waffles.

PREP TIME	COOK TIME	YIELD	DISCARD
10 min (+ overnight rest)	25 minutes	6 waffles	Medium to tangy

INGREDIENTS

1 cup (240 g) sourdough discard, cold
1 cup (90 g) old-fashioned rolled oats (not quick oats)
1 cup (120 g) all-purpose flour
1 tablespoon (12 g) brown sugar
1 teaspoon (4 g) baking powder
½ teaspoon (3 g) baking soda
½ teaspoon (3 g) fine salt

½ teaspoon (1 g) ground cinnamon
2 large eggs
¾ cup (180 ml) whole milk
4 tablespoons (57 g) unsalted butter, melted
1 teaspoon (5 ml) pure vanilla extract

INSTRUCTIONS

1. The night before: Combine the sourdough discard and rolled oats in a medium bowl. Stir well, cover with plastic wrap or a plate, and refrigerate overnight. The oats will absorb the discard and swell considerably.
2. In the morning: Remove the oat mixture from the refrigerator. In a large bowl, whisk together the flour, brown sugar, baking powder, baking soda, salt, and cinnamon.
3. Add the eggs, milk, melted butter, and vanilla to the oat-discard mixture and stir until combined.
4. Pour the wet mixture into the dry ingredients and fold until just combined. The batter will be thick, thicker than a standard waffle batter. That is correct.
5. Cook in a preheated, greased waffle iron as directed in Recipe 04. These waffles may need an extra minute of cook time due to the denser batter.
6. Storage: Refrigerate cooked waffles up to 3 days. Freeze up to 2 months. The uncooked batter can be refrigerated overnight a second time if needed, though the oats will continue to absorb moisture, thin with a tablespoon of milk before cooking if the batter seems very stiff.

Nutritional Information (per waffle)

Calories	Protein	Carbs	Fat	Fiber	Sodium
310	9 g	40 g	12 g	3 g	330 mg

MUFFINS & QUICK BREADS

Muffins and quick breads are among the most forgiving things you can make with sourdough discard. The chemical leaveners do the heavy lifting. The discard contributes flavor, moisture, and a subtle tenderness from its acidity. And unlike pancakes, which need to be eaten immediately, muffins and quick breads keep well for two to three days at room temperature and freeze beautifully.

06 MASTER SOURDOUGH MUFFIN BATTER

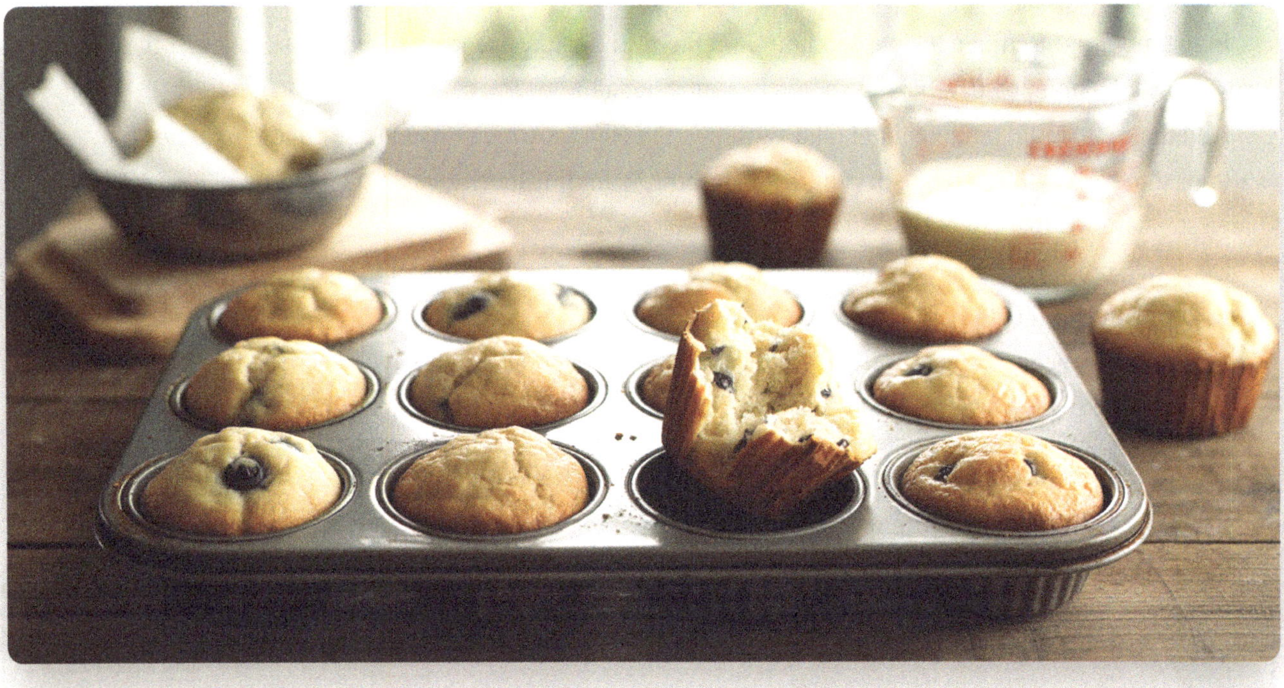

Learn this one formula and you have a dozen muffin recipes. The base batter is neutral enough to take almost any mix-in, fruit, chocolate, nuts, cheese, vegetables, and the discard adds just enough complexity to make it interesting without making it taste like sourdough. Four variations follow.

PREP TIME	COOK TIME	YIELD	DISCARD
12 minutes	20–22 minutes	12 standard muffins	Mild to medium

BASE BATTER INGREDIENTS

2 cups (240 g) all-purpose flour
½ cup (100 g) granulated sugar
2 teaspoons (9 g) baking powder
½ teaspoon (3 g) baking soda
½ teaspoon (3 g) fine salt
¾ cup (180 g) sourdough discard, cold
2 large eggs
⅓ cup (80 ml) whole milk
⅓ cup (75 ml) neutral oil (vegetable or canola)
1 teaspoon (5 ml) pure vanilla extract
1½ cups mix-ins of your choice (see variations below)

INSTRUCTIONS

1. Preheat oven to 375°F (190°C). Line a 12-cup muffin tin with paper liners or grease well with butter and flour.
2. In a large bowl, whisk together the flour, sugar, baking powder, baking soda, and salt.
3. In a medium bowl, whisk together the sourdough discard, eggs, milk, oil, and vanilla until smooth.
4. Pour the wet ingredients into the dry and fold with a spatula until just combined, twelve to fifteen strokes maximum. The batter will look rough and lumpy. This is correct. Overmixed muffins develop tunnels inside and a tough, peaked top.
5. Fold in your chosen mix-ins with two or three additional strokes.
6. Divide the batter evenly among the muffin cups, each should be about three-quarters full. Bake for 20–22 minutes, until a toothpick inserted in the center comes out with just a few moist crumbs attached (not wet batter).
7. Cool in the tin for 5 minutes, then transfer to a wire rack.

BAKER'S TIP

Fill the muffin cups generously, three-quarters full produces a nicely domed muffin. If you fill to only halfway, you'll get flat tops. If you overfill, the batter will spread across the top of the tin. Three-quarters is the right level.

Four Variations

VARIATION A: BANANA WALNUT MUFFINS

The most-requested discard muffin variation. Ripe bananas and discard have a natural affinity, both bring sweetness and complexity, and together they produce a muffin with more depth than a standard banana muffin.

- Replace the milk with ½ cup (115 g) mashed ripe banana (about 1 large, very ripe banana)
- Reduce sugar to ¼ cup (50 g), the banana provides sweetness
- Add ½ teaspoon (1 g) ground cinnamon to the dry ingredients
- Mix-ins: ¾ cup (85 g) chopped toasted walnuts

Nutritional Information (per muffin)

Calories	Protein	Carbs	Fat	Fiber	Sodium
215	5 g	30 g	9 g	1 g	200 mg

VARIATION B: CHEDDAR JALAPEÑO CORN MUFFINS

Savory, slightly spicy, substantial. These work as a side to soup or chili, or as a standalone breakfast with butter.

- Replace ½ cup of the all-purpose flour with ½ cup (85 g) fine yellow cornmeal
- Omit the sugar and vanilla
- Add ¼ teaspoon (0.5 g) garlic powder and ½ teaspoon (1 g) black pepper to the dry ingredients
- Mix-ins: 1 cup (115 g) shredded sharp cheddar + 2 fresh jalapeños, seeded and finely diced (or 2 tablespoons canned diced green chiles for a milder version)

Nutritional Information (per muffin)

Calories	Protein	Carbs	Fat	Fiber	Sodium
195	7 g	24 g	8 g	1 g	310 mg

VARIATION C: LEMON BLUEBERRY LOAF

This variation produces a quick bread rather than muffins, the same batter baked in a 9x5-inch loaf pan. The extended bake time at a lower temperature produces a more tender, dense crumb and a golden top.

- Add the zest of 2 lemons and 2 tablespoons (30 ml) fresh lemon juice to the wet ingredients
- Mix-ins: 1½ cups (225 g) fresh or frozen blueberries (if frozen, do not thaw)
- Bake in a greased 9x5-inch loaf pan at 350°F (175°C) for 55–65 minutes, until a toothpick comes out clean
- Cool in the pan for 15 minutes before turning out

Nutritional Information (per slice, based on 10 slices)

Calories	Protein	Carbs	Fat	Fiber	Sodium
230	5 g	38 g	7 g	1 g	195 mg

VARIATION D: ZUCCHINI BREAD

Sourdough discard and zucchini are a natural pair, both add moisture without heaviness. This is a genuinely good zucchini bread, not a vehicle for using up vegetables.

- Add ½ teaspoon (1 g) ground cinnamon and ¼ teaspoon (0.5 g) ground nutmeg to the dry ingredients
- Add 1 tablespoon (15 ml) additional oil to the wet ingredients
- Fold in 1½ cups (225 g) grated zucchini, do not squeeze out the moisture; the liquid is needed for the bread
- Bake as a loaf (9x5-inch pan) at 350°F (175°C) for 55–60 minutes

Nutritional Information (per slice, based on 10 slices)

Calories	Protein	Carbs	Fat	Fiber	Sodium
195	5 g	30 g	7 g	1 g	210 mg

Storage: All muffins: room temperature in an airtight container up to 3 days, refrigerator up to 5 days, freezer up to 3 months. Loaves: room temperature wrapped tightly up to 4 days, freezer (wrapped and bagged) up to 3 months. Freeze loaves pre-sliced for easy single-serving thawing.

BREAKFAST SAVORIES

Not every morning calls for something sweet. These three recipes cover the savory side of the breakfast chapter, each one using discard in a different way, and each one genuinely fast.

11 SOURDOUGH DISCARD CREPES

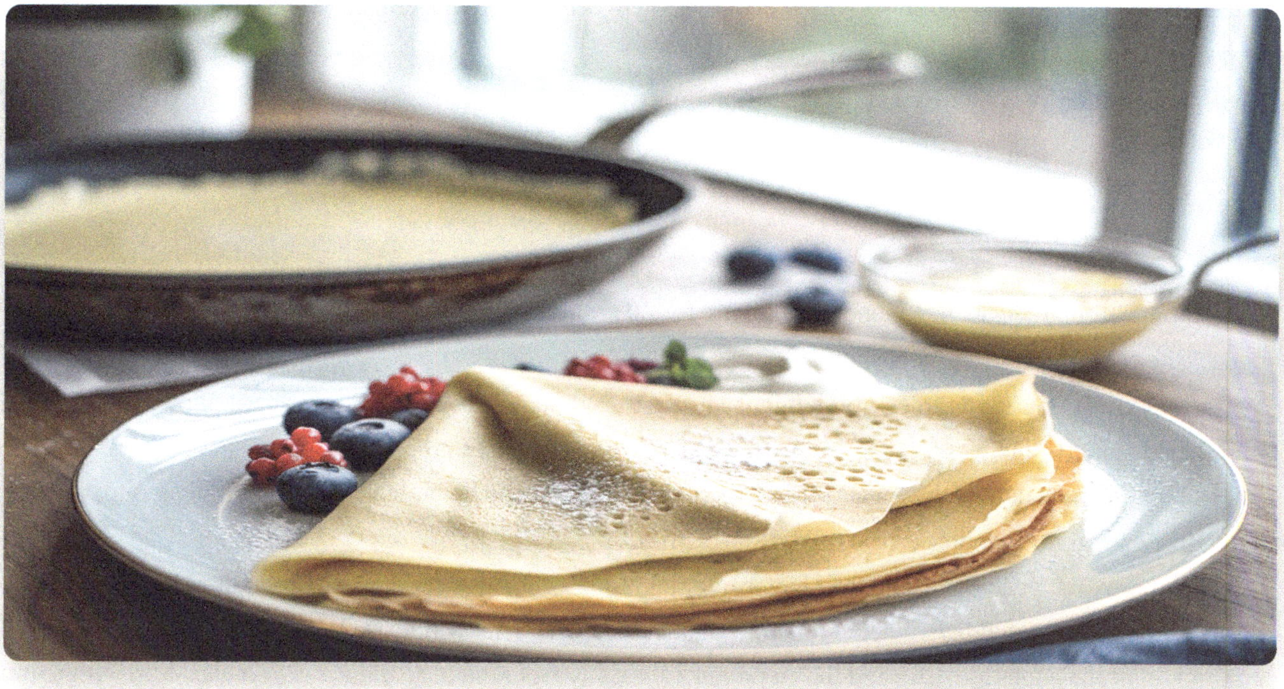

Crepes are the most elegant thing you can make with discard, and also among the easiest. The batter is thinner than pancake batter, the cook time per crepe is under two minutes, and the result is a paper-thin wrapper that works equally well with sweet fillings (jam, Nutella, fresh fruit) or savory ones (ham and cheese, sautéed mushrooms, soft scrambled eggs). Both filling approaches are outlined below.

PREP TIME	**COOK TIME**	**YIELD**	**DISCARD**
5 min (+ 30 min rest)	**20 minutes**	**12–14 crepes**	**Mild**

INGREDIENTS

½ cup (120 g) sourdough discard, cold
¾ cup (90 g) all-purpose flour
2 large eggs
¾ cup (180 ml) whole milk
2 tablespoons (28 g) unsalted butter, melted
1 tablespoon (12 g) granulated sugar (for sweet crepes) OR 1 teaspoon (3 g) fine salt and a pinch of white pepper (for savory crepes)
½ teaspoon (2.5 ml) vanilla extract (sweet version only)

INSTRUCTIONS

1. Combine all ingredients in a blender and blend for 30 seconds until completely smooth. Alternatively, whisk vigorously in a bowl until no lumps remain.
2. Refrigerate the batter for at least 30 minutes and up to 24 hours. This rest is important, it allows the flour to fully hydrate and the bubbles from blending to subside, which produces crepes that don't tear.
3. Heat a 9–10 inch non-stick or well-seasoned crepe pan over medium-high heat. Add a small amount of butter, just enough to coat the surface thinly, and swirl to coat.
4. Pour approximately 3 tablespoons of batter into the center of the pan and immediately tilt and rotate the pan to spread the batter in a thin, even circle. Work quickly, the batter sets within seconds.
5. Cook until the edges look dry and the crepe releases easily from the pan, about 1–2 minutes. Flip with a thin spatula or your fingers and cook for 30 seconds on the second side. The second side will have less even color than the first, this is normal. The first side is the presentation side.
6. Slide onto a plate. Stack crepes directly on top of each other, they will not stick. Continue with remaining batter.
7. Filling Suggestions
8. Sweet: Spread with softened butter and jam, or Nutella and sliced bananas, or lemon curd and fresh berries. Fold in quarters or roll into cylinders.
9. Savory: Fill with thin-sliced ham and gruyère, fold into triangles, and return to the pan briefly to melt the cheese. Or fill with soft scrambled eggs and fresh herbs and roll tightly.

BAKER'S TIP

The first crepe is almost always a throwaway, it calibrates the heat and the fat level in your pan. Eat it in the kitchen and adjust the heat before you make the rest. If crepes are tearing, the batter is too thick (thin with a tablespoon of milk) or the pan is too hot.

Storage: Stacked crepes keep in the refrigerator, covered with plastic wrap, for up to 3 days. Freeze with parchment between each crepe, up to 2 months. Thaw at room temperature for 15 minutes before filling.

Nutritional Information (per crepe, unfilled, based on 13 crepes)

Calories	Protein	Carbs	Fat	Fiber	Sodium
85	3 g	10 g	3 g	0 g	95 mg

12 CRISPY DISCARD HASH BROWNS

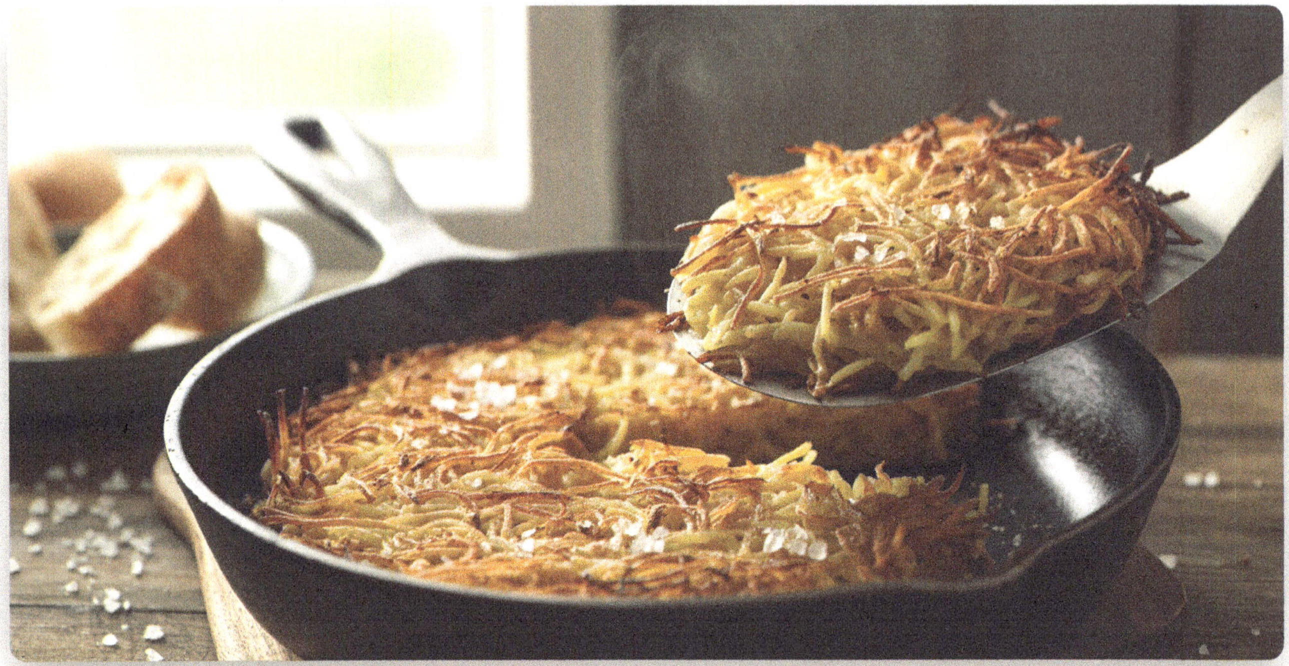

Sourdough discard replaces the egg that traditional hash brown recipes use as a binder, and it does the job better, the acidity helps the starch on the surface of the potato gelatinize faster, which means a crispier exterior in less time. These are genuinely crispy hash browns, not soft, steamed potato cakes.

PREP TIME 15 minutes	COOK TIME 15 minutes	YIELD 4 servings	DISCARD Medium to tangy

INGREDIENTS

2 large russet potatoes (about 600 g / 1.3 lb total), peeled
3 tablespoons (45 g) sourdough discard
½ teaspoon (3 g) fine salt, plus more to taste
¼ teaspoon (0.5 g) freshly ground black pepper
¼ teaspoon (0.5 g) garlic powder
2–3 tablespoons (28–42 g) unsalted butter or clarified butter for frying

INSTRUCTIONS

1. Grate the potatoes on the large holes of a box grater. Transfer to a clean kitchen towel, wrap tightly, and wring out as much moisture as you possibly can. This step is not optional, moisture is the enemy of crispy hash browns. The more liquid you remove, the crispier they will be.
2. In a medium bowl, combine the squeezed potato, sourdough discard, salt, pepper, and garlic powder. Mix until the discard is evenly distributed throughout the potato. The mixture should just hold together when pressed.
3. Heat a large cast iron or heavy-bottomed skillet over medium-high heat. Add the butter and let it melt and foam, when the foam subsides, the butter is ready.
4. Add the potato mixture to the pan in an even layer, pressing down firmly with a spatula. Do not stir or disturb for 5–6 minutes, until the bottom is deep golden brown.
5. Using the spatula, divide into four sections and flip each section carefully. Press down again and cook for another 5–6 minutes until the second side is equally golden.
6. Season with additional salt to taste and serve immediately.

BAKER'S TIP

The most common hash brown mistake is trying to flip too early. The potatoes need time to form a crust before they'll release from the pan cleanly. If they're sticking and tearing when you try to flip, they're not ready. Give them another minute and try again.

Storage: Hash browns are best eaten immediately. Leftovers can be refrigerated up to 2 days and reheated in a dry skillet over medium heat, but they will not be as crispy as fresh.

Nutritional Information (per serving)

Calories	Protein	Carbs	Fat	Fiber	Sodium
210	4 g	32 g	8 g	2 g	305 mg

13 SAVORY BREAKFAST FRITTERS

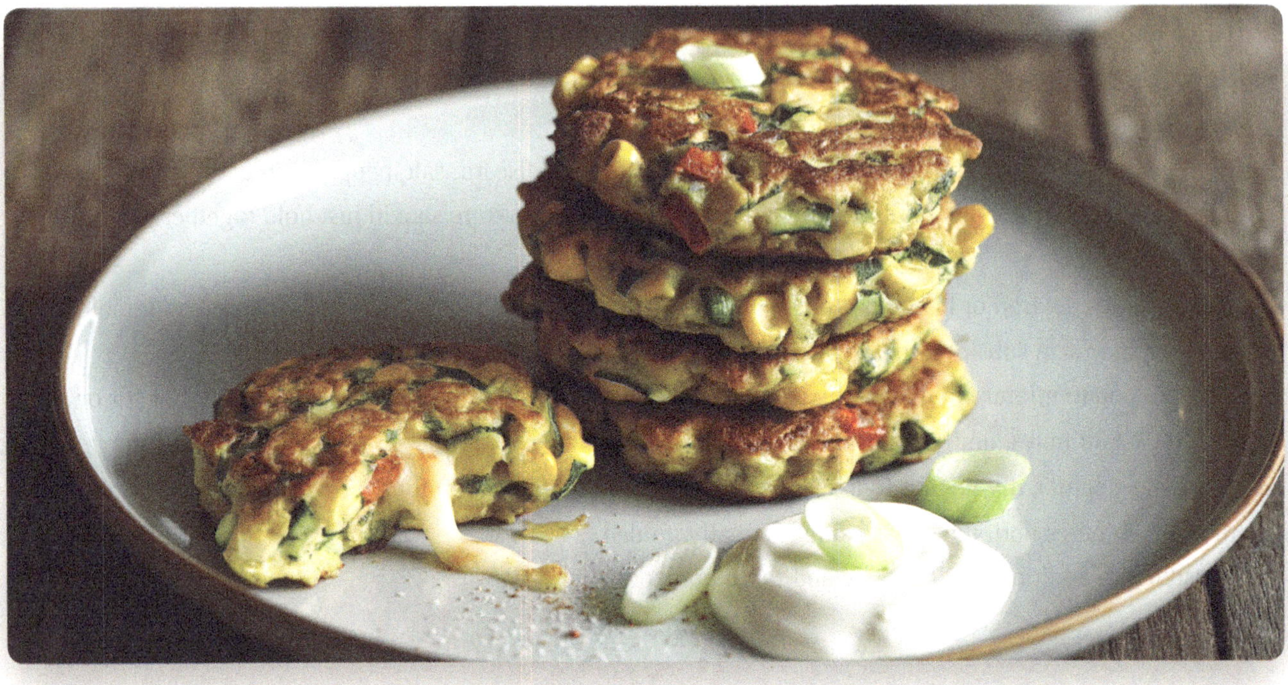

This is the clean-out-the-refrigerator recipe of the breakfast chapter. The base batter holds almost any vegetable or cooked protein you want to add, the list below is a starting point, not a requirement. It is also the most forgiving recipe in this chapter: proportion variations of twenty or thirty percent in either direction will still produce good fritters.

PREP TIME	COOK TIME	YIELD	DISCARD
15 minutes	20 minutes	8–10 fritters	Medium

INGREDIENTS

For the batter:

½ cup (120 g) sourdough discard, cold
½ cup (60 g) all-purpose flour
1 large egg
¼ cup (60 ml) whole milk or water
½ teaspoon (3 g) fine salt
¼ teaspoon (0.5 g) black pepper

½ teaspoon (1 g) your choice of dried herbs (thyme, oregano, or smoked paprika all work well)

For the filling (choose 2–3):

1 cup (about 100 g) grated zucchini, squeezed dry

1 cup (about 90 g) corn kernels, fresh or thawed frozen

½ cup (about 75 g) finely diced red bell pepper

3 scallions, thinly sliced

½ cup (55 g) shredded cheese (cheddar, gruyère, or feta all work)

½ cup (about 75 g) diced cooked ham, bacon, or sausage

INSTRUCTIONS

1. In a large bowl, whisk together the discard, flour, egg, milk, salt, pepper, and dried herbs until a smooth batter forms.
2. Fold in your chosen filling ingredients. The batter will be thick, almost like a dip, and that is correct. It should hold its shape when dropped from a spoon.
3. Heat 2 tablespoons of oil in a large skillet over medium heat. When the oil shimmers, drop heaping tablespoonfuls of the batter into the pan, spacing them about 2 inches apart. Flatten each slightly with the back of the spoon.
4. Cook for 3–4 minutes until the bottom is golden and the edges look set. Flip and cook for another 2–3 minutes until cooked through.
5. Drain briefly on paper towels. Serve with sour cream, hot sauce, or a fried egg on top.
6. Storage: Refrigerate up to 3 days. Reheat in a skillet or 375°F oven for 8 minutes. Freeze up to 2 months; reheat from frozen in a 375°F oven for 12–15 minutes.

Nutritional Information (per fritter, based on 9 fritters with zucchini, corn, and cheddar filling)

Calories	Protein	Carbs	Fat	Fiber	Sodium
145	6 g	17 g	6 g	1 g	285 mg

BISCUITS

Biscuits occupy a category of their own because they are simultaneously one of the simplest and most technically interesting things you can make with discard. The technique is minimal, no mixer, no special equipment, twenty minutes from bowl to oven. But the results are genuinely excellent: tall, flaky, tender biscuits with a subtle tang from the discard and a buttery, crispy bottom.

14 SOURDOUGH DISCARD BISCUITS

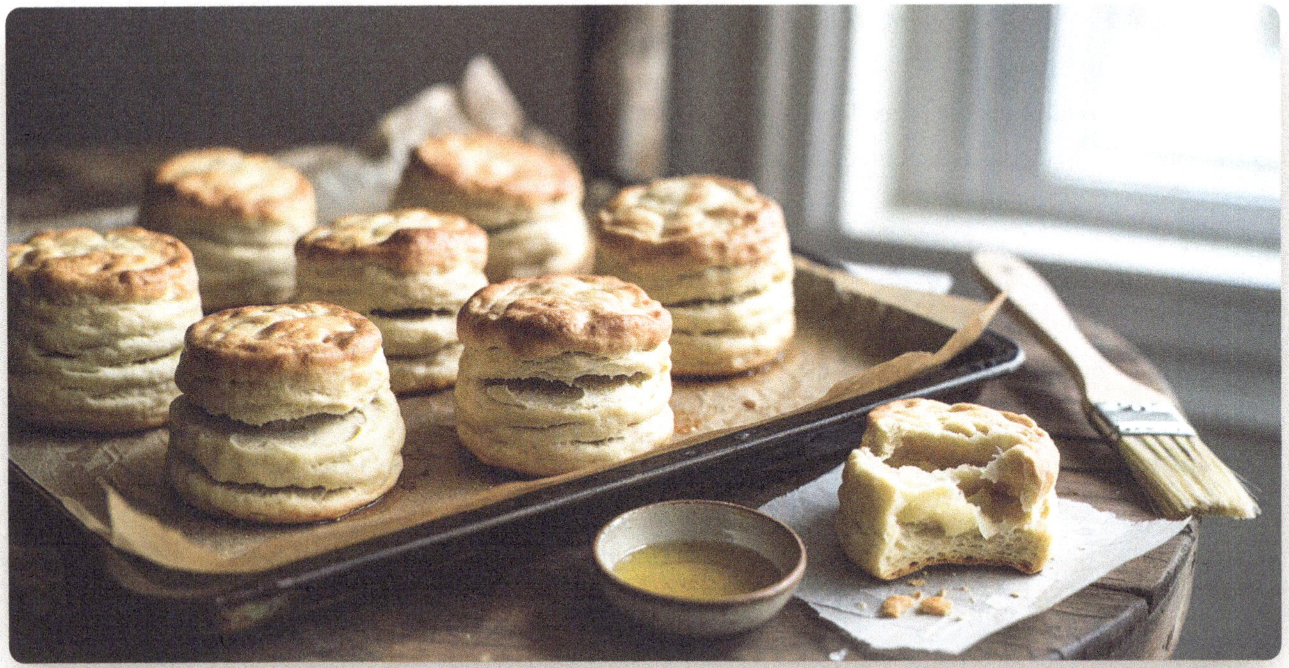

These are flaky, layered, pull-apart biscuits, not cakey drop biscuits. The lamination technique (folding the dough) is what creates the layers, and it takes two minutes. The discard's acidity makes the biscuits more tender than standard biscuits and gives them a flavor that is noticeably more interesting than anything made with commercial buttermilk.

PREP TIME	COOK TIME	YIELD	DISCARD
20 minutes	14–16 minutes	8 biscuits	Medium

INGREDIENTS

2 cups (240 g) all-purpose flour, plus more for dusting
1 tablespoon (12 g) baking powder
½ teaspoon (3 g) baking soda
1 teaspoon (6 g) fine salt
1 teaspoon (4 g) granulated sugar

½ cup (113 g) unsalted butter, very cold, frozen is ideal
½ cup (120 g) sourdough discard, cold
¼ cup (60 ml) whole milk or buttermilk, cold

INSTRUCTIONS

1. Preheat oven to 425°F (220°C). Line a baking sheet with parchment paper.
2. Whisk together the flour, baking powder, baking soda, salt, and sugar in a large bowl.
3. Grate the cold butter directly into the flour mixture using the large holes of a box grater. Toss the butter shreds in the flour with your fingers until each piece is coated. You want visible pieces of butter throughout, this is what creates steam and layers during baking.
4. In a small bowl, stir together the sourdough discard and milk. Pour this mixture into the flour-butter mixture and fold with a spatula or your hands until a shaggy dough just comes together. It will look rough and barely cohesive. That is exactly right.
5. Turn the dough out onto a lightly floured surface. Pat it into a rough rectangle, about ¾ inch thick. Fold the dough in thirds like a letter. Pat flat again. Fold in thirds again. This two-fold lamination creates the layers. Do not overwork the dough, six to eight gentle pats and two folds is all it needs.
6. Pat the final dough to ¾ inch thickness. Cut with a sharp 2½-inch round cutter, press straight down without twisting. Twisting seals the edges and prevents the biscuits from rising straight up. Place on the prepared baking sheet with sides just touching.
7. Bake for 14–16 minutes until the tops are deep golden brown. Brush with melted butter the moment they come out of the oven.

BAKER'S TIP

Cold butter is non-negotiable for flaky biscuits. If your kitchen is warm and the butter softens while you're working, put the entire mixing bowl in the freezer for 10 minutes before continuing. The visible chunks of butter in the dough melt during baking, releasing steam that pushes the layers apart. If the butter melts before it gets in the oven, that steam never happens and you get dense biscuits instead of flaky ones.

Storage: Room temperature in an airtight container up to 2 days. Refrigerate up to 4 days. Freeze (pre-baked) up to 3 months, reheat from frozen in a 350°F oven for 12 minutes. You can also freeze the unbaked cut biscuits and bake directly from frozen; add 4–5 minutes to the bake time.

Nutritional Information (per biscuit)

Calories	Protein	Carbs	Fat	Fiber	Sodium
245	5 g	30 g	12 g	1 g	390 mg

CHAPTER 4

Crackers & Flatbreads

Crackers are the most underrated thing you can make with sourdough discard, and this chapter is going to change how you think about them.

The usual perception of homemade crackers is that they're a novelty, something impressive to bring to a party, but not something you'd make regularly because it takes too much effort. That perception is based on experience with recipes that are unnecessarily complicated. The crackers in this chapter are not complicated. The master recipe requires six ingredients, fifteen minutes of active work, and produces results that are categorically better than anything you can buy in a box.

Discard is ideal for crackers for a simple reason: crackers don't need to rise. The limitations that matter in yeasted bread, discard's reduced leavening power, are completely irrelevant here. What crackers need is flavor, structure, and the right ratio of fat to starch for crispness. Discard provides all three. Its acidity also works with the baking process to produce crackers that stay crispy longer than crackers made without it.

Flatbreads follow naturally from crackers, they use similar techniques and similar ingredients, but with more thickness and a softer, more pliable result. All of the flatbreads in this chapter are same-day recipes: no overnight rise, no advance planning, nothing that requires you to have thought ahead.

> *Crackers are the one category where older, more assertively sour discard actually performs better than mild discard. The tang stands up to bold toppings and gives the cracker a flavor that plain flour and water cannot replicate.*

One technical note before the recipes: thickness is the most important variable in cracker baking. A cracker that is one millimeter too thick will be tough and chewy rather than crispy. A cracker that is too thin will burn before it crisps. Every recipe in this chapter specifies thickness, take it seriously. Roll between two sheets of parchment with a consistent, even pressure, and check the thickness by holding the dough up to the light before it goes in the oven. You'll know quickly if one area is thicker than the rest.

CRACKERS

15 MASTER THIN SOURDOUGH CRACKER

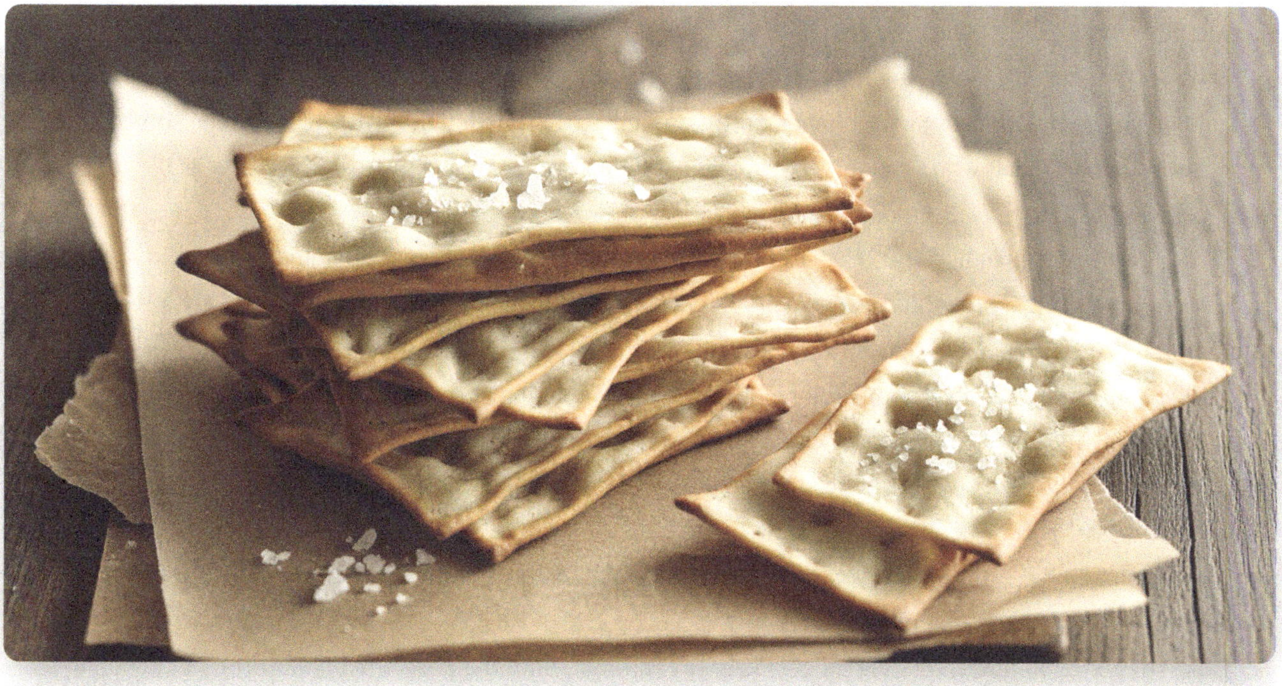

This is the foundation recipe for everything in the cracker section. Learn this one and you can make any of the variations that follow by changing only the toppings and seasonings. The dough is simple, forgiving, and produces a cracker that is genuinely crispy, not hard, not tough, but the clean, light snap of a well-made thin cracker.

PREP TIME 15 minutes	COOK TIME 18–22 minutes	YIELD About 60 crackers	DISCARD Medium to tangy

INGREDIENTS

1 cup (240 g) sourdough discard, cold

1 cup (120 g) all-purpose flour, plus more for dusting

3 tablespoons (42 g) unsalted butter, melted, or 3 tablespoons (45 ml) olive oil

½ teaspoon (3 g) fine salt, plus flaky salt for topping

½ teaspoon (1 g) your choice of dried herb or spice (see variations below)

1 tablespoon (15 ml) water, if needed

INSTRUCTIONS

1. Preheat oven to 325°F (165°C). This lower temperature is deliberate, it dries the crackers out evenly without burning the edges before the center crisps.
2. In a medium bowl, combine the sourdough discard, flour, melted butter or olive oil, salt, and your chosen seasoning. Mix with a spatula or your hands until a smooth, cohesive dough forms. It should be soft but not sticky. If it's crumbly and won't come together, add water one teaspoon at a time until it holds. If it's sticking to your hands, add flour one tablespoon at a time.
3. Divide the dough in half. Place one half between two sheets of parchment paper and roll as thin as you can, aim for 1–2 mm, roughly the thickness of a credit card. If the dough springs back as you roll, let it rest for 3 minutes and try again. Gluten relaxes quickly.
4. Slide the parchment with the rolled dough directly onto a baking sheet. Peel off the top sheet of parchment. Score the dough into your desired cracker shape with a pizza cutter or sharp knife, squares, rectangles, or irregular shards all work. You do not need to separate the pieces before baking; they'll break apart cleanly along the scored lines after they cool.
5. Spray or brush the surface lightly with water and sprinkle with flaky salt and any additional toppings. Press toppings in gently so they adhere.
6. Bake for 18–22 minutes, rotating the pan halfway through, until the crackers are uniformly golden and feel dry to the touch. The edges will color faster than the center, this is normal. Watch for the center to lose its pale, raw look. If individual crackers on the edges are getting too dark before the center is done, remove those pieces and return the rest to the oven.
7. Cool completely on the pan. The crackers will continue to crisp as they cool, do not judge them until they are fully at room temperature, at least 15 minutes after coming out of the oven.

BAKER'S TIP

The most common cracker mistake is pulling them too early. A cracker that looks slightly underdone at 20 minutes will often be perfect once cool. A cracker that goes back in for 3 more minutes because it looked pale will frequently be right. If your crackers are soft after cooling, they needed more time, return them to a 300°F oven for 8–10 more minutes, cool again, and they will crisp.

Storage: Airtight container at room temperature up to 1 week. Do not refrigerate, the humidity will soften them. They do not freeze well. If they soften over time, crisp them in a 300°F oven for 5 minutes and cool completely before serving.

Nutritional Information (per cracker, based on 60 crackers)

Calories	Protein	Carbs	Fat	Fiber	Sodium
18	0 g	3 g	1 g	0 g	30 mg

Three Seasoning Variations

Each variation uses the Master Thin Cracker dough as its base. Only the toppings and any additions to the dough change.

- Plain & Seeded: Mix 2 tablespoons (18 g) sesame seeds and 1 tablespoon (9 g) poppy seeds into the dough. Top with flaky salt only.
- Herbed: Add 1 teaspoon (1 g) dried rosemary and ½ teaspoon (0.5 g) dried thyme to the dough. Top with flaky salt and a few additional fresh rosemary leaves pressed in lightly.
- Spiced: Add ½ teaspoon (1 g) smoked paprika, ½ teaspoon (1 g) cumin, and a pinch of cayenne to the dough. Top with flaky salt. These are excellent with hummus or a sharp cheese.

16 EVERYTHING BAGEL CRACKERS

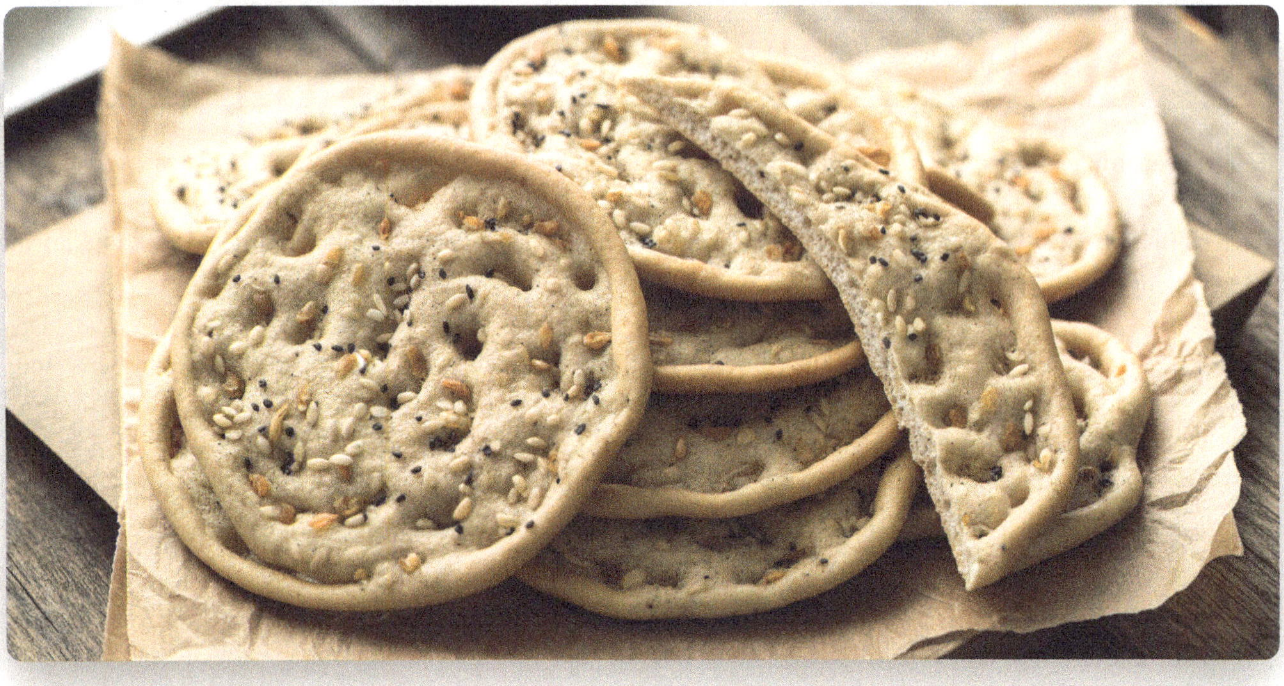

Everything bagel seasoning and sourdough discard are a natural pairing, both have complexity and umami depth that reinforce each other. These crackers taste significantly better than everything bagel chips from a store, and they take about the same amount of effort as opening a bag.

PREP TIME 15 minutes	COOK TIME 20–24 minutes	YIELD About 55 crackers	DISCARD Medium

INGREDIENTS

1 cup (240 g) sourdough discard, cold
1 cup (120 g) all-purpose flour
2 tablespoons (28 g) unsalted butter, melted
1 tablespoon (15 ml) olive oil
½ teaspoon (3 g) fine salt
1 large egg white, beaten (for wash)
3 tablespoons (27 g) everything bagel seasoning (store-bought or homemade: equal parts sesame seeds, poppy seeds, dried garlic flakes, dried onion flakes, and flaky salt)

INSTRUCTIONS

1. Preheat oven to 325°F (165°C). In a medium bowl, mix together the discard, flour, melted butter, olive oil, and salt until a smooth dough forms.
2. Divide in half and roll each half between parchment sheets to 1–2 mm thickness. Slide onto baking sheets, peel off the top parchment, and score into desired shapes.
3. Brush the surface lightly with beaten egg white, this is the adhesive that makes the seasoning stick through baking. Sprinkle generously with everything bagel seasoning and press in gently.
4. Bake for 20–24 minutes, rotating halfway, until evenly golden. The garlic and onion in the seasoning will color faster than plain crackers, watch for the difference between golden and burnt. Cool completely before breaking apart.

BAKER'S TIP

Everything bagel seasoning is very salty. Taste your seasoning before applying, some commercial blends are saltier than others. If yours is heavily salted, omit the fine salt from the dough or reduce it to ¼ teaspoon.

Storage: Airtight container at room temperature up to 1 week.

Nutritional Information (per cracker, based on 55 crackers)

Calories	Protein	Carbs	Fat	Fiber	Sodium
20	1 g	3 g	1 g	0 g	55 mg

17 PARMESAN ROSEMARY CRACKERS

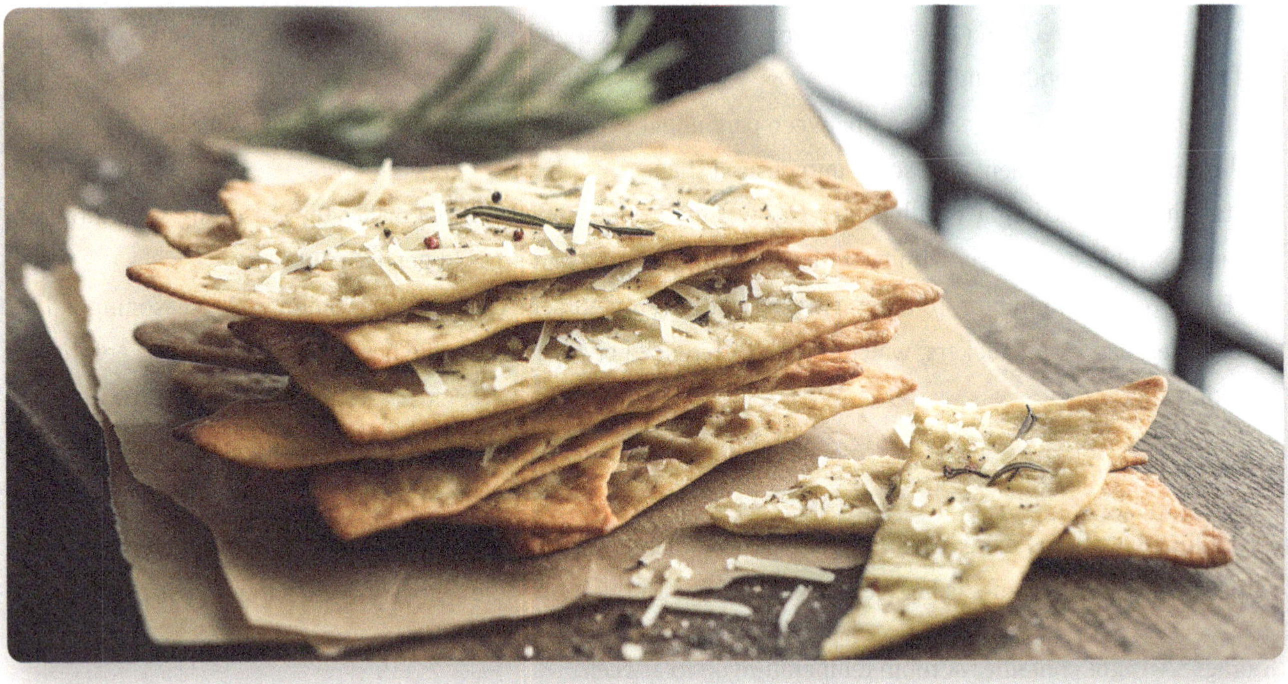

These are the crackers you make when you want something that looks and tastes like it came from a specialty food shop. The parmesan bakes into the cracker itself rather than sitting on top, which means every bite has cheese flavor throughout, not just on the surface.

PREP TIME 15 minutes	COOK TIME 20–24 minutes	YIELD About 50 crackers	DISCARD Mild to medium

INGREDIENTS

1 cup (240 g) sourdough discard, cold
¾ cup (90 g) all-purpose flour
¼ cup (25 g) fine semolina flour (or substitute all-purpose, semolina adds snap)
½ cup (50 g) finely grated Parmesan, divided
3 tablespoons (42 g) unsalted butter, melted
2 teaspoons (2 g) finely chopped fresh rosemary (or 1 tsp dried)
½ teaspoon (3 g) fine salt
¼ teaspoon (0.5 g) freshly ground black pepper

INSTRUCTIONS

1. Preheat oven to 325°F (165°C). Combine the discard, all-purpose flour, semolina, ¼ cup of the Parmesan (reserve the rest for topping), butter, rosemary, salt, and pepper. Mix until a smooth dough forms.
2. Divide in half, roll each half to 1–2 mm between parchment, slide onto baking sheets, and score into crackers. Sprinkle the remaining ¼ cup of Parmesan over the surface and press in lightly.
3. Bake 20–24 minutes until deep golden, the cheese on top will color faster than the cracker body. Cool completely before breaking apart.

BAKER'S TIP

Use the finest grater setting for the Parmesan that goes into the dough, it needs to fully incorporate. For the topping, slightly coarser grating creates better texture and visual appeal.

Storage: Airtight container at room temperature up to 5 days. The cheese makes these slightly more perishable than plain crackers.

Nutritional Information (per cracker, based on 50 crackers)

Calories	Protein	Carbs	Fat	Fiber	Sodium
22	1 g	3 g	1 g	0 g	45 mg

18 RYE DISCARD CRISPBREADS

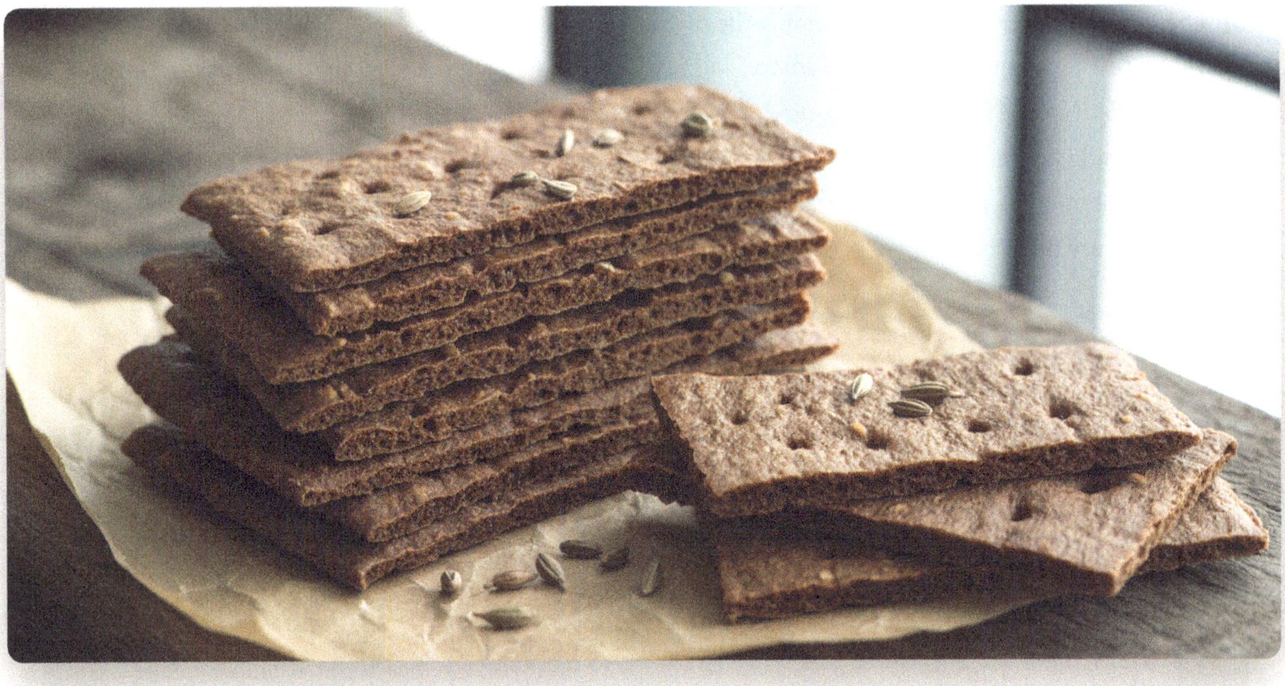

Scandinavian-style crispbreads are thicker than thin crackers but still fully crispy, more like a dense, snapping wafer than a cracker. They are designed for older, more assertively sour discard; the rye flour amplifies the tang in a way that is intentional and very good. Top with smoked salmon and cream cheese, or simply with butter and a pinch of salt.

PREP TIME 15 minutes	COOK TIME 25–30 minutes	YIELD About 20 crispbreads	DISCARD Tangy

INGREDIENTS

½ cup (120 g) sourdough discard, cold, older and tangier is better here
½ cup (60 g) dark rye flour
½ cup (60 g) all-purpose flour
2 tablespoons (30 ml) olive oil
½ teaspoon (3 g) fine salt
¼ teaspoon (0.5 g) caraway seeds (optional but traditional)
3–4 tablespoons (45–60 ml) cold water, added gradually
Flaky salt and additional caraway or sesame seeds for topping

INSTRUCTIONS

1. Preheat oven to 350°F (175°C), slightly higher than thin crackers because these are thicker and need more heat to dry through.
2. Combine the discard, rye flour, all-purpose flour, olive oil, salt, and caraway if using. Mix until crumbly, then add cold water one tablespoon at a time until the dough just comes together. Rye dough is stickier and less elastic than all-purpose dough, this is normal.
3. Roll the dough between parchment to about 3 mm thickness, thicker than thin crackers, thinner than a flatbread. The surface will be slightly rougher and less smooth than white flour dough; don't try to make it perfect.
4. Score into rectangles approximately 3 x 5 inches, or use a fork to dock (prick) the surface all over, which prevents puffing. Sprinkle with flaky salt and additional seeds.
5. Bake 25–30 minutes until firm and dry throughout, rotating halfway. These take longer than thin crackers because of their thickness. They should sound hollow when tapped lightly on the bottom. Cool completely on the pan.

BAKER'S TIP

Rye flour absorbs water more slowly than all-purpose flour. If the dough seems very dry after mixing, wait two minutes before adding more water, the rye is still hydrating. Add water gradually; rye dough that's too wet becomes sticky and difficult to roll.

Storage: Airtight container at room temperature up to 2 weeks. These keep better than thin crackers and actually improve in flavor over the first few days.

Nutritional Information (per crispbread, based on 20 pieces)

Calories	Protein	Carbs	Fat	Fiber	Sodium
65	2 g	11 g	2 g	1 g	95 mg

19 SESAME MISO CRACKERS

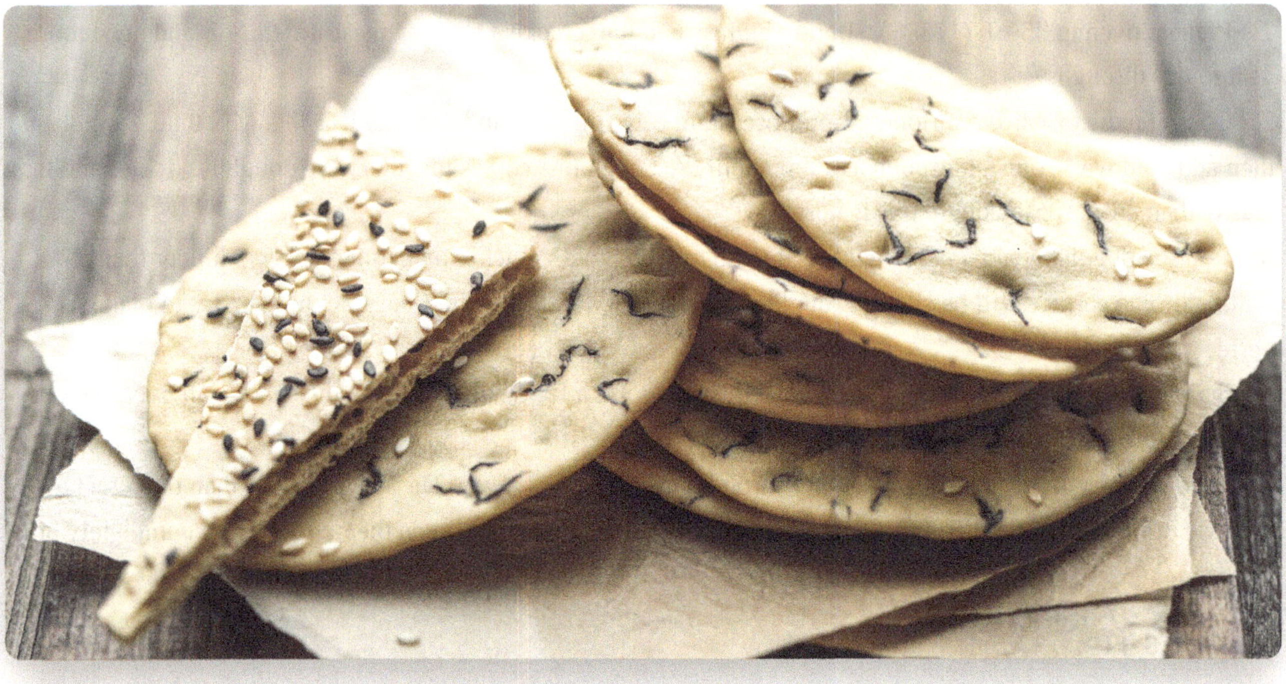

Miso paste in a cracker dough sounds unusual until you taste the result: a deep, savory, slightly sweet complexity that has nothing to do with tasting like miso soup. The white or yellow miso available at most grocery stores works perfectly here. These pair particularly well with sharp cheddar, aged gouda, or a soft fresh cheese.

PREP TIME 15 minutes	COOK TIME 20–24 minutes	YIELD About 55 crackers	DISCARD Mild to medium

INGREDIENTS

1 cup (240 g) sourdough discard, cold
1 cup (120 g) all-purpose flour
2 tablespoons (30 g) white or yellow miso paste
2 tablespoons (28 g) unsalted butter, melted
1 tablespoon (15 ml) sesame oil (toasted)
¼ cup (36 g) sesame seeds (white, black, or a mix), divided
No additional salt, the miso provides enough

INSTRUCTIONS

1. Preheat oven to 325°F (165°C). Whisk together the discard and miso until fully smooth, miso can form lumps if not fully incorporated, and those lumps will burn during baking.
2. Add the flour, melted butter, sesame oil, and half the sesame seeds. Mix until a smooth dough forms.
3. Roll to 1–2 mm between parchment, slide onto baking sheets, score into shapes, and sprinkle with the remaining sesame seeds. Press in gently.
4. Bake 20–24 minutes until golden. Watch carefully, the miso causes slightly faster browning than plain dough. Cool completely before breaking.

Storage: Airtight container at room temperature up to 1 week.

Nutritional Information (per cracker, based on 55 crackers)

Calories	Protein	Carbs	Fat	Fiber	Sodium
21	1 g	3 g	1 g	0 g	40 mg

20 GRAHAM-STYLE CRACKERS

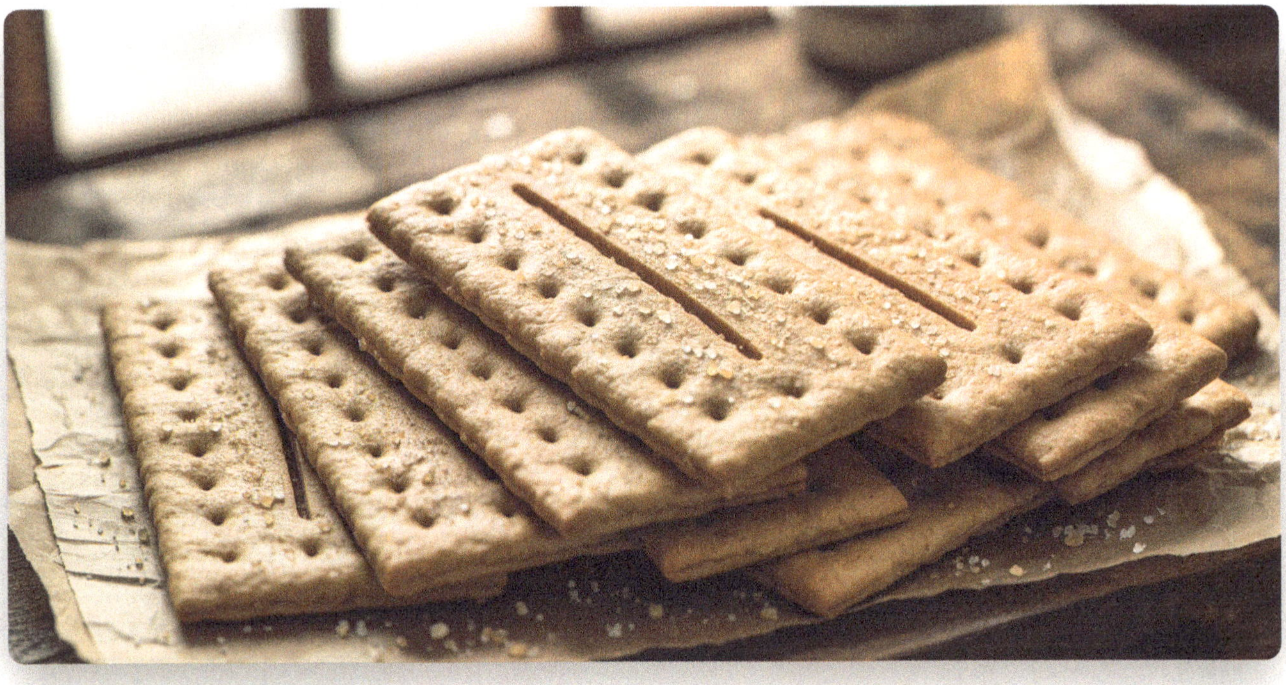

These occupy the space between sweet and savory, slightly honeyed, warmly spiced, with the tang of discard giving them more complexity than a standard graham cracker. They work as a snack on their own, as a base for a dessert crust (press into a tart pan with butter), or as a vehicle for peanut butter and sliced banana.

PREP TIME 15 minutes	**COOK TIME** 18–20 minutes	**YIELD About** 40 crackers	**DISCARD** Mild

INGREDIENTS

¾ cup (180 g) sourdough discard, cold
¾ cup (90 g) all-purpose flour
½ cup (60 g) whole wheat flour
3 tablespoons (63 g) honey
2 tablespoons (28 g) unsalted butter, melted
1 teaspoon (2 g) ground cinnamon
½ teaspoon (3 g) fine salt
¼ teaspoon (1 g) baking soda

Turbinado or coarse sugar for topping

INSTRUCTIONS

1. Preheat oven to 325°F (165°C). Combine all ingredients except the topping sugar and mix until a smooth dough forms. The whole wheat flour makes this dough slightly stiffer than the master cracker dough, this is normal.
2. Roll to 2 mm thickness between parchment. Score into rectangles, traditional graham crackers are about 2.5 x 5 inches, and press a fork pattern down the center of each one for the classic look. Sprinkle with turbinado sugar and press lightly.
3. Bake 18–20 minutes until firm and dry, with lightly golden edges. Cool completely, these continue crisping as they cool more than other crackers do.

BAKER'S TIP

For a crispier cracker, reduce the honey to 2 tablespoons. More honey makes a slightly chewier, more cookie-like cracker. Both are good, it depends on what you want them for. For a dessert crust, the chewier version holds together better when pressed into a pan.

Storage: Airtight container at room temperature up to 1 week. For use as a crust, do not pre-bake the crust, press the raw cracker dough directly into a pan and bake the whole tart together.

Nutritional Information (per cracker, based on 40 crackers)

Calories	Protein	Carbs	Fat	Fiber	Sodium
35	1 g	6 g	1 g	0 g	40 mg

FLATBREADS

Flatbreads are crackers grown up, thicker, softer, with enough body to fold, wrap, or top generously. All four of the flatbreads in this chapter are same-day recipes that require no yeast and no rise time. They go from mixing bowl to table in under forty-five minutes, and they are substantially better than store-bought pita or tortillas in a way that surprises people every time.

21 SAME-DAY DISCARD FLATBREAD

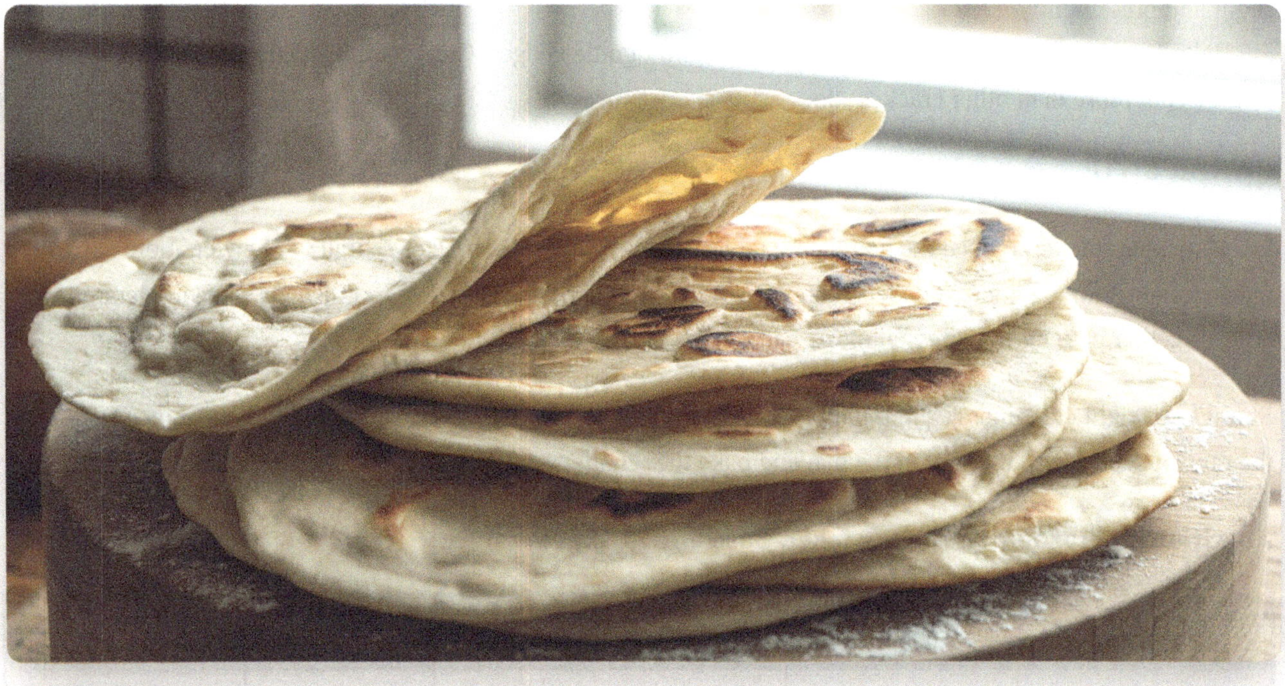

This is the workhorse flatbread recipe, the one you'll make so often it becomes automatic. Six ingredients, no rise time, ready in thirty minutes. It works as a wrap, a pizza base, a dipping vehicle for hummus, or a side bread alongside soup or salad. The discard gives it a slight chew and a flavor that plain flour flatbreads don't have.

PREP TIME	COOK TIME	YIELD	DISCARD
10 minutes	15 minutes	6 flatbreads	Mild to medium

INGREDIENTS

1 cup (240 g) sourdough discard, cold

1 cup (120 g) all-purpose flour, plus more for dusting
1 tablespoon (15 ml) olive oil
½ teaspoon (3 g) fine salt
½ teaspoon (4 g) baking powder
2 tablespoons (30 ml) plain yogurt (optional, adds tenderness and a slight tang)

INSTRUCTIONS

1. In a medium bowl, combine the discard, flour, olive oil, salt, and baking powder. Add the yogurt if using. Mix until a soft, slightly tacky dough forms. If it's very sticky, add flour one tablespoon at a time. If it's stiff and cracking, add water one teaspoon at a time.
2. Divide the dough into 6 equal pieces. On a lightly floured surface, roll each piece into a thin oval or circle, about 6–7 inches across and 3–4 mm thick. Don't aim for perfect circles, irregular edges are part of the charm of a handmade flatbread.
3. Heat a dry cast iron skillet or heavy-bottomed pan over medium-high heat until very hot, a drop of water should evaporate instantly on contact. No oil is needed.
4. Cook each flatbread for 1½–2 minutes per side, until dark spots appear on the surface and the flatbread puffs slightly in places. The puffing is good, it means steam is trapped between layers, which is what creates a soft, pliable interior.
5. Stack cooked flatbreads and cover with a clean towel as you work, the steam keeps them soft and pliable.

BAKER'S TIP

The key to flatbreads that puff and stay soft is a very hot pan and quick cooking. A pan that isn't hot enough produces pale, dense flatbreads that don't puff. If your flatbreads aren't developing dark spots within 90 seconds on the first side, increase the heat.

Storage: Room temperature, wrapped in a towel or foil, up to 1 day, they are best eaten the day they are made. Refrigerate in an airtight container up to 3 days; reheat in a dry skillet for 30 seconds per side to restore softness. Freeze up to 2 months with parchment between each piece.

Nutritional Information (per flatbread)

Calories	Protein	Carbs	Fat	Fiber	Sodium
140	4 g	26 g	3 g	1 g	200 mg

22 DISCARD PIZZA DOUGH

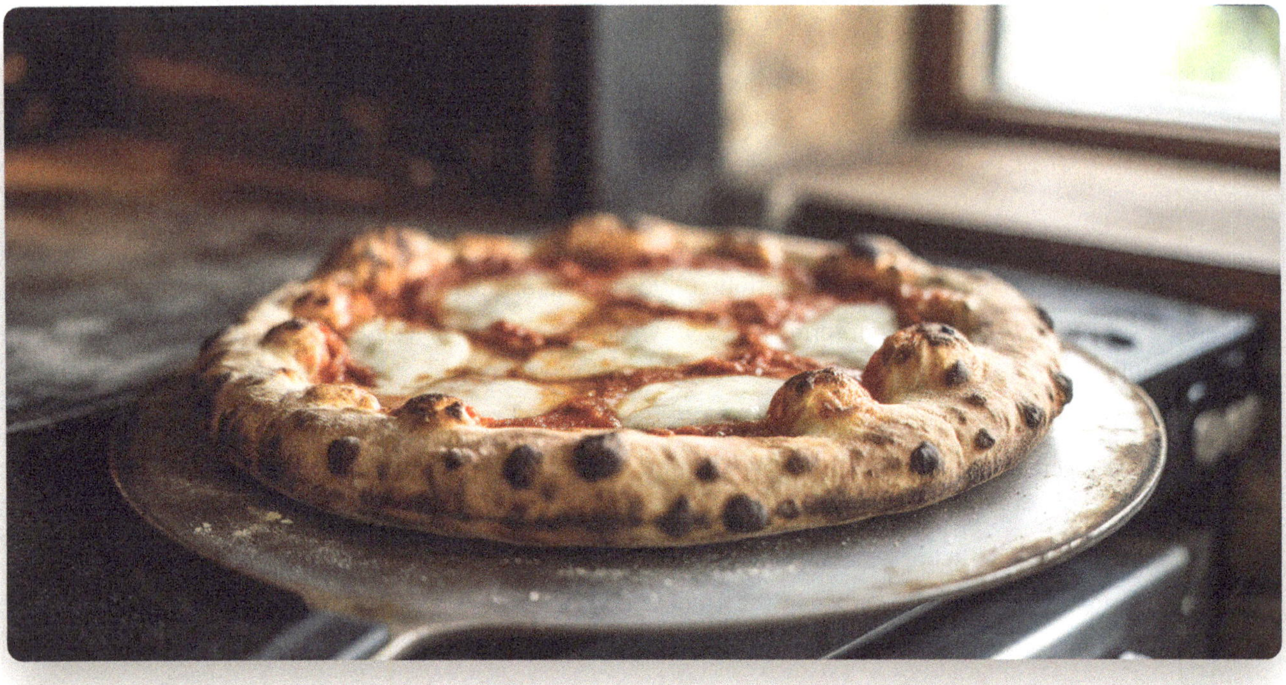

This produces a real pizza dough, not a flatbread dressed up as pizza, but a properly chewy, slightly charred crust with a crumb that has some structure to it. The discard contributes flavor that compressed yeast can't produce, and because you're using baking powder as a backup leavener, you don't need to wait for a rise. Same-day pizza with better flavor than most yeasted versions.

PREP TIME	COOK TIME	YIELD	DISCARD
15 minutes	12–15 minutes	2 pizzas (10–12 inch)	Medium

INGREDIENTS

¾ cup (180 g) sourdough discard, cold
1½ cups (180 g) all-purpose flour, plus more for shaping
1 teaspoon (5 g) baking powder
½ teaspoon (3 g) fine salt
1 teaspoon (4 g) granulated sugar
2 tablespoons (30 ml) olive oil
3–5 tablespoons (45–75 ml) cold water, added gradually

INSTRUCTIONS

1. Place a baking sheet or pizza stone in the oven and preheat to 475°F (245°C) for at least 30 minutes. The hot surface is what gives the bottom of the crust its crispness.
2. In a large bowl, whisk together the flour, baking powder, salt, and sugar. Add the discard, olive oil, and 3 tablespoons of water. Mix until a shaggy dough forms, then knead briefly in the bowl, about 2 minutes, until smooth. Add additional water one tablespoon at a time if the dough seems dry.
3. Divide in half. On a lightly floured surface, stretch or roll each piece into a 10–12 inch round. For thin crust: roll to 3 mm. For thick crust: leave it at 5–6 mm. The dough will resist stretching at first, let it rest for 5 minutes and try again.
4. Transfer to a piece of parchment paper. Add sauce and toppings. Slide the parchment directly onto the hot baking surface.
5. Bake thin crust for 10–12 minutes, thick crust for 13–15 minutes, until the cheese is bubbling and the edges of the crust are deep golden brown.

BAKER'S TIP

For the crispiest possible bottom crust, remove the parchment after the first 5 minutes of baking, carefully slide it out from under the pizza using tongs. The direct contact with the hot pan surface for the final minutes of baking produces significant additional crispness.

Storage: Unbaked dough can be refrigerated, wrapped tightly, up to 2 days, the additional fermentation time actually improves the flavor. Bring to room temperature for 30 minutes before shaping. Baked pizza keeps refrigerated up to 3 days; reheat in a 375°F oven for 8 minutes or in a dry skillet over medium-low heat with a lid on for 5 minutes.

Nutritional Information (per serving, based on ¼ of one pizza)

Calories	Protein	Carbs	Fat	Fiber	Sodium
310	9 g	52 g	8 g	2 g	380 mg

23 PITA-STYLE DISCARD BREAD

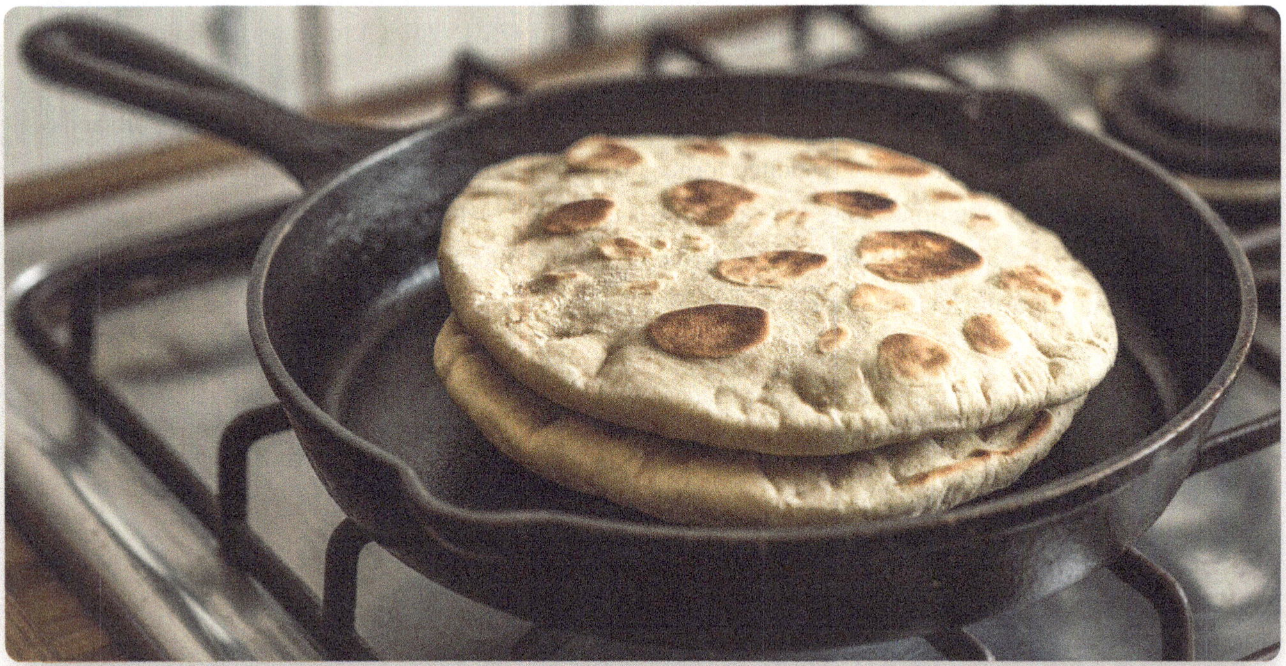

This is one of the most satisfying things to make in the cast iron pan. Discard pita puffs dramatically into a hollow pocket as it hits the hot surface, the steam inside expands the dough before the structure sets. The result is a proper pita with a real pocket, made in under ten minutes of active time and without a single packet of yeast.

PREP TIME	COOK TIME	YIELD	DISCARD
15 min (+ 20 min rest)	20 minutes	6 pitas	Mild to medium

INGREDIENTS

¾ cup (180 g) sourdough discard, cold
1¼ cups (150 g) all-purpose flour, plus more for dusting
1 teaspoon (5 g) baking powder
½ teaspoon (3 g) fine salt
1 tablespoon (15 ml) olive oil
¼ cup (60 ml) warm water

INSTRUCTIONS

1. Combine the discard, flour, baking powder, salt, olive oil, and warm water in a bowl. Mix until a soft dough forms, then knead on a lightly floured surface for 3–4 minutes until smooth and elastic. The dough should be soft but not sticky, add flour by the teaspoon if it sticks.
2. Cover the dough with a bowl or plastic wrap and rest at room temperature for 20 minutes. This rest is important: it allows the gluten to relax so the dough rolls thin without springing back, and it gives the baking powder time to activate slightly, which helps puffing.
3. Divide the dough into 6 equal pieces. Roll each into a thin circle, about 6 inches across and 3–4 mm thick. Try to keep an even thickness throughout, thin spots puff, thick spots don't.
4. Heat a dry cast iron or heavy-bottomed skillet over high heat until very hot. Cook each pita for 1½–2 minutes on the first side, the surface will bubble and the edges will start to look dry. Flip and cook for another minute. The pita may puff dramatically on the second side; this is the goal.
5. Transfer to a plate and cover immediately with a clean towel. The steam trapped inside keeps the pita soft and pliable.

BAKER'S TIP

If your pitas aren't puffing: the pan isn't hot enough, or the dough is too thick. A very hot pan is essential, the rapid heat causes the steam inside to expand faster than the dough can set, creating the pocket. If pitas consistently don't puff, try rolling them slightly thinner.

Storage: Cool completely before storing. Room temperature in a sealed bag up to 2 days. Refrigerate up to 5 days; warm in a dry skillet or microwave with a damp paper towel for 20 seconds before serving. Freeze up to 3 months.

Nutritional Information (per pita)

Calories	Protein	Carbs	Fat	Fiber	Sodium
165	5 g	30 g	3 g	1 g	225 mg

24 SOCCA-STYLE CHICKPEA FLATBREAD

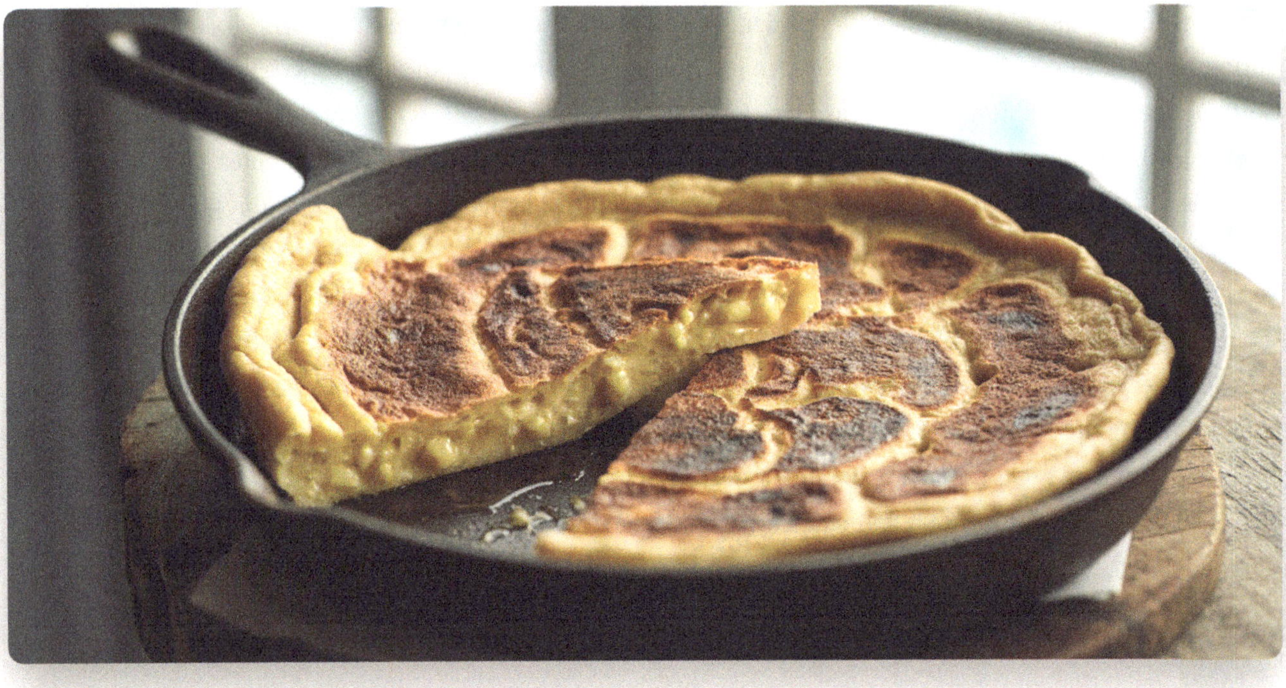

Socca is a traditional Provençal street food made from chickpea flour, olive oil, and water, cooked in a screaming hot cast iron pan until it develops a crispy exterior and a custardy, almost creamy interior. Adding sourdough discard to the batter deepens the flavor considerably and helps the flatbread set more evenly. This is naturally gluten-light (not gluten-free, the small amount of discard contains gluten), dairy-free, and done in twenty minutes.

PREP TIME	COOK TIME	YIELD	DISCARD
5 min (+ 30 min rest)	15 minutes	2 large flatbreads (4 servings)	Medium

INGREDIENTS

1 cup (100 g) chickpea flour (also sold as besan or gram flour)
¼ cup (60 g) sourdough discard, cold
¾ cup (180 ml) warm water
3 tablespoons (45 ml) olive oil, divided
½ teaspoon (3 g) fine salt
¼ teaspoon (0.5 g) freshly ground black pepper

Optional additions: 1 teaspoon fresh rosemary, finely chopped; 2 tablespoons caramelized onions; a pinch of smoked paprika

INSTRUCTIONS

1. Whisk together the chickpea flour, discard, warm water, 2 tablespoons of the olive oil, salt, and pepper until completely smooth. Add any optional ingredients. Rest the batter at room temperature for 30 minutes, chickpea flour needs time to fully hydrate.
2. Position an oven rack in the upper third of the oven and preheat the broiler to high. Place a 10–12 inch cast iron skillet under the broiler to heat for 5 minutes.
3. Carefully remove the hot skillet from the oven. Add the remaining 1 tablespoon of olive oil and swirl to coat. Pour in half the batter and swirl to create an even, thin layer.
4. Return to the broiler for 4–6 minutes, until the top is set and developing dark spots and the edges are pulling away from the pan slightly. The center should be firm when the pan is gently shaken.
5. Slide onto a cutting board and cut into wedges. Repeat with the remaining batter.

BAKER'S TIP

The broiler method is essential for socca, it provides high, direct heat from above that creates the characteristic blistered, charred top while keeping the inside slightly creamy. A stovetop method works but produces a less interesting result. Watch it carefully under the broiler; the difference between perfectly charred and burnt is about 90 seconds.

Storage: Best eaten immediately. Leftovers can be refrigerated up to 2 days and reheated in a hot skillet for 2 minutes per side, though the texture changes somewhat. Does not freeze well.

Nutritional Information (per serving, based on 4 servings)

Calories	Protein	Carbs	Fat	Fiber	Sodium
195	8 g	20 g	10 g	3 g	310 mg

CHAPTER 5

Sweet Bakes and Desserts

People are often surprised to learn that sourdough discard belongs in desserts. The assumption is that sour and sweet are opposites that cancel each other out, and that adding discard to a chocolate cake will produce something that tastes like sourdough bread masquerading as dessert.

That assumption is wrong, and the chemistry explains why.

In sweet recipes, sugar suppresses the perception of acidity. Fat coats the palate and softens sharp flavors. Vanilla, chocolate, cinnamon, and fruit each have enough aromatic intensity to redirect attention away from the discard's tang entirely. What remains after these ingredients do their work is not sourness. It is complexity. A chocolate cake made with sourdough discard has a deeper, more interesting flavor than the same cake without it. Cookies have more chew. Quick breads have a more tender crumb. The discard is working underneath the surface, not announcing itself.

There is one situation where tang becomes noticeable in sweet recipes: when the discard is very old and assertively sour, and the recipe is relatively light in sugar and fat. Delicate recipes like shortbread or crepes are more sensitive to sour discard than rich recipes like brownies or chocolate cake. The discard profile column in each recipe's meta bar tells you which level of sourness works best.

> *The discard is not the flavor in these recipes. It is the thing that makes the other flavors more interesting. That is a meaningful distinction, and it is why these desserts convert skeptics.*

The ten recipes in this chapter move from cakes to cookies and bars to pastry and special occasion bakes. Each one has been chosen because it demonstrates something specific about what discard does in a sweet context.

CAKES

25 SOURDOUGH CHOCOLATE CAKE

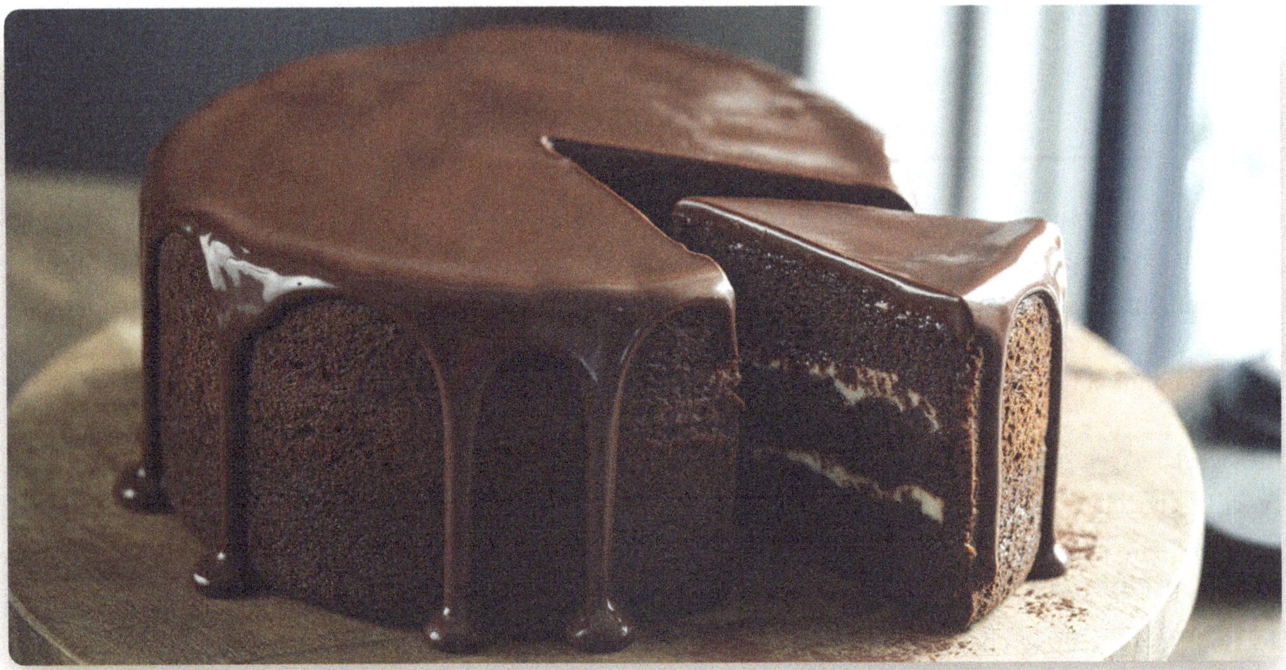

This is the showstopper. It is deeply chocolatey, fudgy without being dense, and has a complexity of flavor that standard chocolate cakes made with commercial leaveners do not achieve. The discard contributes acidity that reacts with the cocoa powder (an alkali) to deepen the chocolate flavor and darken the crumb. No one who eats this cake will taste sourdough. They will simply taste a very good chocolate cake and want another slice.

PREP TIME 20 minutes	COOK TIME 35 minutes	YIELD One 9-inch round cake (12 slices)	DISCARD Mild to medium

INGREDIENTS

For the cake:

1 cup (240 g) sourdough discard, cold

1 cup (120 g) all-purpose flour

1 cup (200 g) granulated sugar

3/4 cup (75 g) unsweetened cocoa powder (Dutch-process preferred)
1 teaspoon (5 g) baking soda
1/2 teaspoon (2 g) baking powder
1/2 teaspoon (3 g) fine salt
2 large eggs, room temperature
1/2 cup (120 ml) whole milk
1/2 cup (120 ml) neutral oil (vegetable or canola)
1 teaspoon (5 ml) pure vanilla extract
1/2 cup (120 ml) hot coffee or hot water (coffee deepens the chocolate flavor)
For the frosting (simple ganache):
1 cup (170 g) dark chocolate chips or finely chopped dark chocolate
1/2 cup (120 ml) heavy cream
1 tablespoon (14 g) unsalted butter
Pinch of fine salt

INSTRUCTIONS

1. Preheat oven to 350 degrees F (175 degrees C). Grease a 9-inch round cake pan and line the bottom with a parchment circle. Grease the parchment.
2. In a large bowl, whisk together the flour, sugar, cocoa powder, baking soda, baking powder, and salt until fully combined and no cocoa lumps remain.
3. In a separate bowl, whisk together the sourdough discard, eggs, milk, oil, and vanilla until smooth.
4. Pour the wet ingredients into the dry and stir until just combined. Add the hot coffee or water and stir again until the batter is smooth. The batter will be thin. This is correct.
5. Pour into the prepared pan and bake for 32 to 36 minutes, until a toothpick inserted in the center comes out with just a few moist crumbs. Do not overbake. This cake is meant to be slightly fudgy in the center when fully cooked.
6. Cool in the pan for 15 minutes, then turn out onto a wire rack to cool completely before frosting.
7. For the ganache: heat the cream in a small saucepan until it just begins to simmer. Pour over the chocolate chips in a heatproof bowl. Let sit for 2 minutes without stirring, then add the butter and salt and stir from the center outward until completely smooth and glossy. Let the ganache cool for 20 to 30 minutes until it thickens slightly before spreading over the cooled cake.

BAKER'S TIP

Dutch-process cocoa produces a darker, smoother, less acidic chocolate flavor than natural cocoa. If you only have natural cocoa, the cake will still be good but slightly lighter in color and with a slightly sharper chocolate bite. Do not substitute hot chocolate mix or sweetened cocoa.

Storage: Room temperature under a cake dome up to 2 days. Refrigerate up to 5 days; bring to room temperature before serving. Freeze unfrosted cake layers (wrapped tightly) up to 3 months.

Nutritional Information (per slice, based on 12 slices, with ganache)

Calories	Protein	Carbs	Fat	Fiber	Sodium
385	6 g	52 g	19 g	3 g	290 mg

26 BROWN BUTTER BANANA CAKE

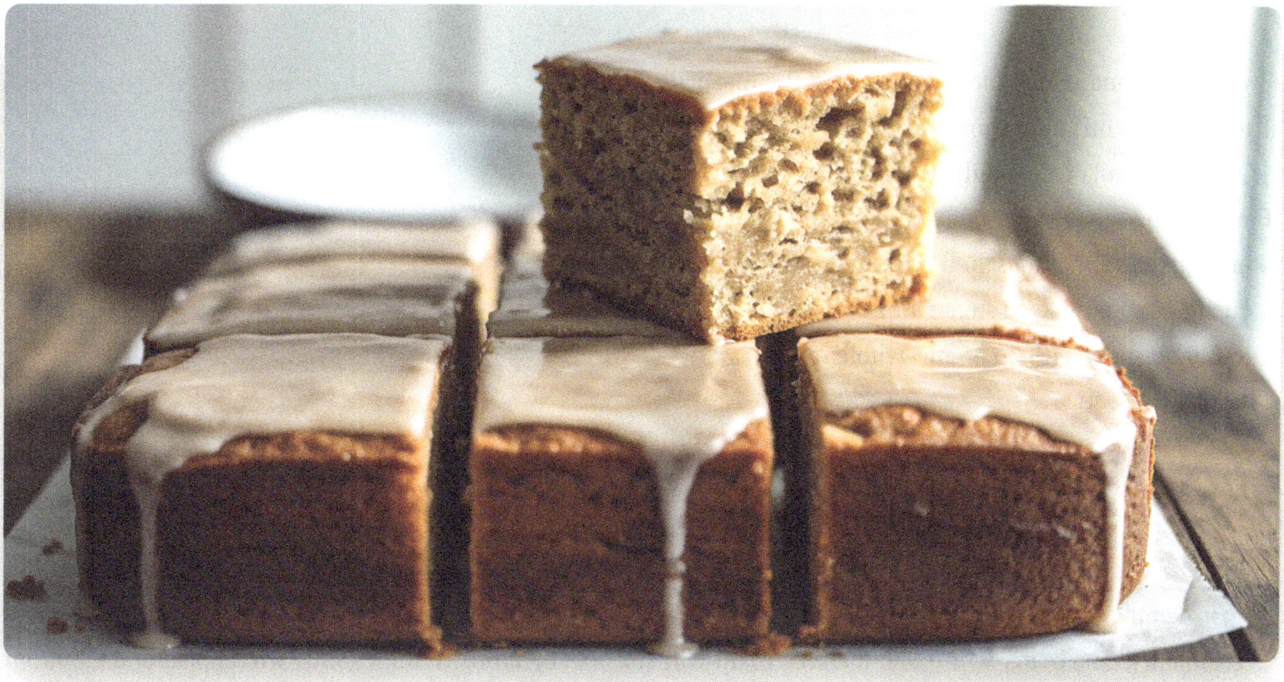

Brown butter and overripe bananas are each individually excellent. Together with sourdough discard, they produce a cake that is more complex than any banana bread or banana cake you have made before. The browned milk solids add a nutty, caramel-like depth. The discard extends the banana flavor and adds a slight tang that keeps the cake from being cloying. This is not a quick bread baked in a cake pan. It is a genuinely different thing.

PREP TIME	COOK TIME	YIELD One	DISCARD
20 minutes	35 minutes	9 x 13-inch cake (16 slices)	Mild

INGREDIENTS

For the cake:

1/2 cup (113 g) unsalted butter

3/4 cup (180 g) sourdough discard, cold

1 1/2 cups (180 g) all-purpose flour

1 teaspoon (4 g) baking powder

1/2 teaspoon (3 g) baking soda

1/2 teaspoon (3 g) fine salt

1 teaspoon (2 g) ground cinnamon
3/4 cup (150 g) granulated sugar
1/4 cup (55 g) packed brown sugar
2 large eggs
3 very ripe bananas (about 1 1/4 cups / 300 g mashed)
1 teaspoon (5 ml) pure vanilla extract
1/2 cup (120 ml) whole milk
For the brown butter glaze:
4 tablespoons (57 g) unsalted butter
1 cup (120 g) powdered sugar, sifted
2 to 3 tablespoons (30 to 45 ml) whole milk
Pinch of fine salt

INSTRUCTIONS

1. Brown the butter first: melt the 1/2 cup butter in a light-colored saucepan over medium heat. Swirl occasionally. The butter will foam, then the foam will subside, then brown milk solids will appear at the bottom and the butter will smell nutty and toasted. This takes 5 to 7 minutes. Pour immediately into a large mixing bowl to stop the cooking and cool for 10 minutes.
2. Preheat oven to 350 degrees F (175 degrees C). Grease a 9x13-inch baking pan.
3. In a medium bowl, whisk together the flour, baking powder, baking soda, salt, and cinnamon.
4. Add both sugars to the cooled brown butter and whisk until combined. Add the eggs one at a time, whisking well after each. Add the mashed bananas, sourdough discard, vanilla, and milk and stir until smooth.
5. Fold the dry ingredients into the wet ingredients until just combined. Pour into the prepared pan and smooth the top.
6. Bake for 32 to 36 minutes until the top is set and a toothpick comes out clean. Cool completely in the pan before glazing.
7. For the glaze: brown the 4 tablespoons butter as described above. Whisk in the powdered sugar, milk, and salt until smooth and pourable. Drizzle over the cooled cake.

BAKER'S TIP

Browning butter is fast once it starts. Do not walk away during the final 2 minutes. The difference between perfectly browned and burnt is about 30 seconds. If you smell anything acrid rather than nutty, pour it immediately into the bowl even if it looks lighter than expected.

Storage: Room temperature covered up to 3 days. Refrigerate up to 5 days. Freeze unglazed in individual slices up to 2 months.

Nutritional Information (per slice, based on 16 slices, with glaze)

Calories	Protein	Carbs	Fat	Fiber	Sodium
265	4 g	38 g	11 g	1 g	175 mg

27 OLIVE OIL CITRUS CAKE

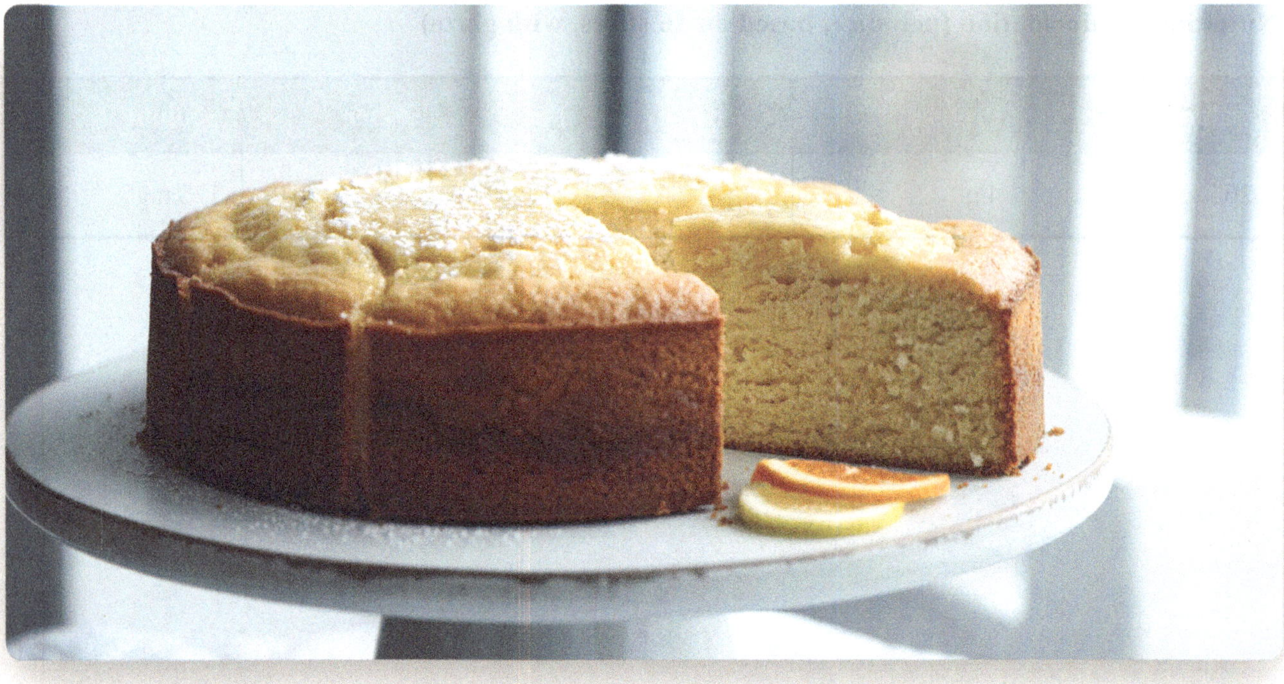

This is the simplest cake in the chapter and also one of the most elegant. It requires no mixer, no special technique, and produces a moist, tender crumb with a bright citrus flavor and a subtle richness from the olive oil that butter cannot replicate. The discard adds a very gentle tang that plays perfectly against the lemon and orange. Serve it with whipped cream and fresh berries, or simply dusted with powdered sugar.

PREP TIME 15 minutes	**COOK TIME 40 minutes**	**YIELD One 9-inch round cake (10 slices)**	**DISCARD Mild**

INGREDIENTS

3/4 cup (180 g) sourdough discard, cold
1 1/2 cups (180 g) all-purpose flour
1 cup (200 g) granulated sugar
1 1/2 teaspoons (6 g) baking powder
1/2 teaspoon (3 g) fine salt
3 large eggs
3/4 cup (180 ml) good-quality olive oil (not extra-virgin, which can be bitter)

1/4 cup (60 ml) whole milk
Zest of 1 large lemon
Zest of 1 orange
2 tablespoons (30 ml) fresh lemon juice
Powdered sugar for dusting

INSTRUCTIONS

1. Preheat oven to 350 degrees F (175 degrees C). Grease a 9-inch round cake pan and line with parchment.
2. In a large bowl, whisk together the flour, sugar, baking powder, and salt.
3. In a separate bowl, whisk together the eggs, olive oil, milk, sourdough discard, lemon zest, orange zest, and lemon juice until smooth.
4. Pour the wet ingredients into the dry and whisk until smooth. This batter is less sensitive to overmixing than most cake batters because olive oil cakes have no gluten development concern at this ratio.
5. Pour into the prepared pan and bake for 38 to 42 minutes, until the top is deep golden and a toothpick comes out clean. The cake will pull slightly away from the sides of the pan when done.
6. Cool in the pan for 20 minutes, then unmold onto a rack. Dust generously with powdered sugar before serving.

BAKER'S TIP

This cake improves significantly the day after baking. The olive oil and discard continue to moisten the crumb as it rests, and the citrus flavor deepens. If you can make it the night before serving, do.

Storage: Covered at room temperature up to 3 days. Refrigerate up to 5 days. Freeze (without powdered sugar) up to 2 months.

Nutritional Information (per slice, based on 10 slices)

Calories	Protein	Carbs	Fat	Fiber	Sodium
320	5 g	38 g	17 g	1 g	195 mg

COOKIES AND BARS

Discard performs differently in cookies than in cakes. In cakes, it adds moisture and flavor while staying mostly invisible. In cookies, its acidity interacts with butter and sugar in a way that affects texture directly: more chew, slightly denser centers, better spread control. The four recipes below each demonstrate a different aspect of this effect.

28 CHEWY CHOCOLATE CHIP COOKIES

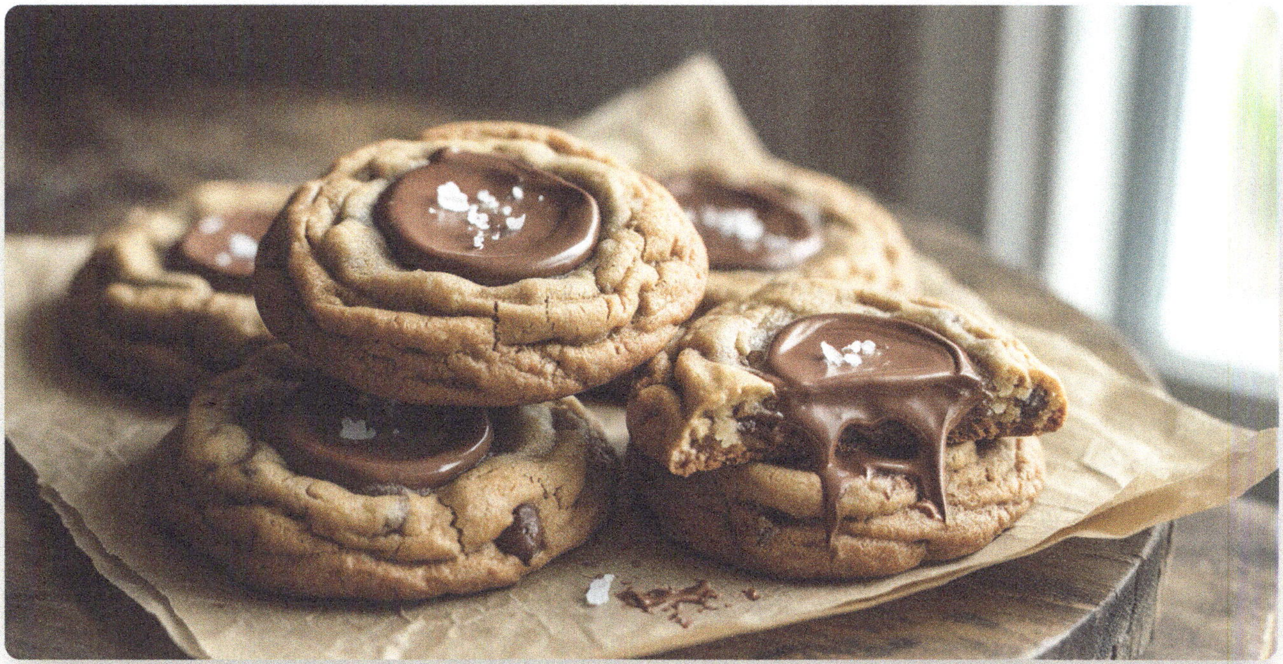

These are chewy in the best possible way: set at the edges, soft in the center, with a slight resistance that holds up for two days rather than going either crunchy or completely soft by the next morning. The discard is doing two things here: the acidity slows the spread of the cookie during baking (producing a thicker, chewier result), and it adds a flavor note that makes the chocolate taste more complex without making the cookie taste remotely like sourdough.

PREP TIME	COOK TIME	YIELD	DISCARD
15 min (+ 1 hour chill)	12 minutes	24 cookies	Mild to medium

INGREDIENTS

1/2 cup (120 g) sourdough discard, cold
2 cups (240 g) all-purpose flour
1 teaspoon (4 g) baking soda
1 teaspoon (6 g) fine salt
3/4 cup (170 g) unsalted butter, softened to room temperature
3/4 cup (150 g) granulated sugar
3/4 cup (165 g) packed brown sugar

2 large eggs
2 teaspoons (10 ml) pure vanilla extract
2 cups (340 g) semi-sweet chocolate chips
Flaky salt for topping

INSTRUCTIONS

1. In a medium bowl, whisk together the flour, baking soda, and salt. Set aside.
2. In a large bowl, beat the softened butter with both sugars until light and fluffy, about 3 minutes with a hand mixer or 5 minutes by hand. Add the eggs one at a time, mixing well after each addition. Add the vanilla and sourdough discard and mix until fully incorporated.
3. Add the flour mixture and fold with a spatula until just combined. Fold in the chocolate chips.
4. Cover the bowl and refrigerate for at least 1 hour and up to 72 hours. The chilling is important: it firms the butter, which controls spread during baking and improves flavor through additional fermentation of the discard. Longer chilling produces noticeably better cookies.
5. When ready to bake, preheat oven to 375 degrees F (190 degrees C). Line baking sheets with parchment.
6. Scoop balls of dough approximately 2 tablespoons each onto the prepared sheets, spacing about 2 inches apart. Sprinkle with flaky salt.
7. Bake for 10 to 12 minutes until the edges are set and golden but the centers still look underdone and shiny. They will firm up as they cool. Remove from the oven and let cool on the baking sheet for 5 minutes before transferring.

BAKER'S TIP

Pull these cookies when they still look slightly underdone in the center. The residual heat from the baking sheet will finish them over the next 5 minutes. A cookie that looks perfectly done in the oven will be overbaked and dry once cool. Trust the underdone appearance.

Storage: Airtight container at room temperature up to 4 days. Freeze baked cookies up to 2 months. Alternatively, freeze the unbaked scooped dough balls and bake directly from frozen, adding 2 to 3 minutes to the bake time.

Nutritional Information (per cookie, based on 24 cookies)

Calories	Protein	Carbs	Fat	Fiber	Sodium
195	3 g	27 g	9 g	1 g	145 mg

29 SNICKERDOODLES

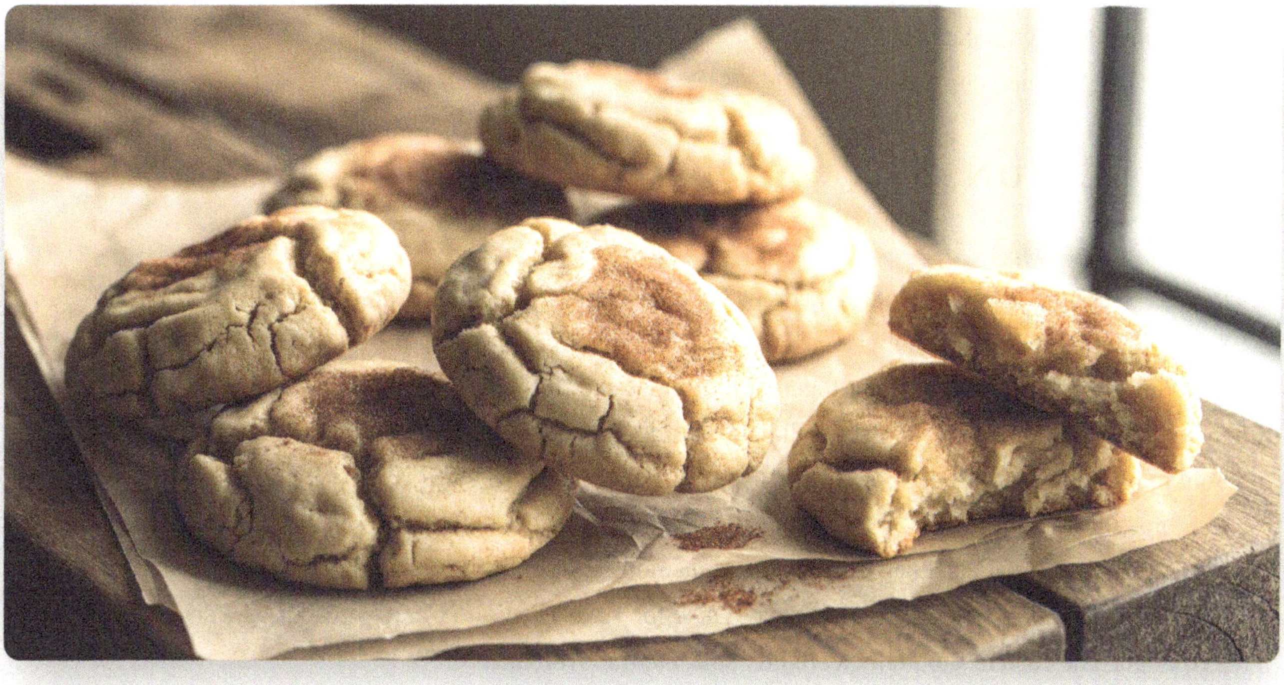

Classic snickerdoodles rely on cream of tartar for their signature tang and chewy texture. Sourdough discard provides both of these things naturally, which means this recipe produces a better snickerdoodle than the traditional version while using an ingredient you already have. The cinnamon sugar coating crisps slightly during baking and then softens as the cookie cools, producing the characteristic crinkled, slightly crunchy exterior.

PREP TIME	COOK TIME	YIELD	DISCARD
15 minutes	11 minutes	30 cookies	Mild

INGREDIENTS

For the dough:
1/2 cup (120 g) sourdough discard, cold
2 3/4 cups (330 g) all-purpose flour
1 teaspoon (4 g) baking soda
1/2 teaspoon (3 g) fine salt
1 cup (226 g) unsalted butter, softened
1 1/2 cups (300 g) granulated sugar

2 large eggs

1 teaspoon (5 ml) pure vanilla extract

For the coating:

3 tablespoons (36 g) granulated sugar

2 teaspoons (4 g) ground cinnamon

INSTRUCTIONS

1. Preheat oven to 375 degrees F (190 degrees C). Line baking sheets with parchment.
2. Whisk together the flour, baking soda, and salt in a medium bowl.
3. Beat the softened butter and sugar together until light and fluffy, about 3 minutes. Add the eggs one at a time, mixing well after each. Add the vanilla and sourdough discard and mix until smooth.
4. Fold in the flour mixture until just combined.
5. Combine the coating sugar and cinnamon in a small shallow bowl. Scoop dough into balls of about 1.5 tablespoons each and roll each ball through the cinnamon sugar until fully coated.
6. Place on the prepared sheets 2 inches apart. Bake for 10 to 11 minutes until the edges are set and the tops have crinkled. The centers should look slightly soft. Do not overbake.
7. Cool on the baking sheet for 5 minutes before transferring.

BAKER'S TIP

For a more pronounced tang that plays against the cinnamon sugar, use medium discard (4 to 7 days old) rather than fresh mild discard. The contrast between the sour cookie base and the sweet coating is what makes a great snickerdoodle, and slightly older discard amplifies that contrast naturally.

Storage: Airtight container at room temperature up to 5 days. Freeze baked cookies or unbaked dough balls up to 2 months.

Nutritional Information (per cookie, based on 30 cookies)

Calories	Protein	Carbs	Fat	Fiber	Sodium
155	2 g	22 g	7 g	0 g	80 mg

30 FUDGY SOURDOUGH BROWNIES

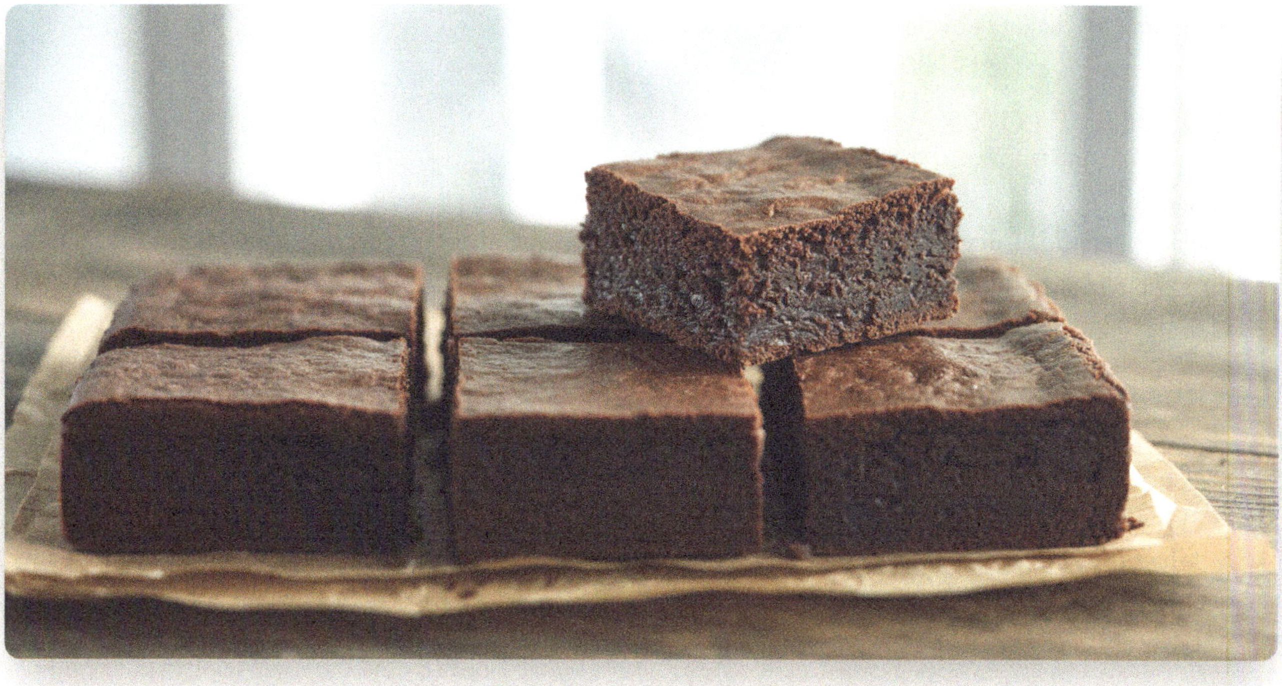

The discard's role in these brownies is purely textural. The acidity tenderizes the gluten in the flour and interacts with the baking powder to produce a crumb that is denser and moister than standard brownies without being gluey. You will not taste it. You will simply eat a better brownie and not know why. These are fudgy-style brownies rather than cakey: dense centers, slightly crisp tops, and a clean snap when cut cold.

PREP TIME	COOK TIME	YIELD	DISCARD
15 minutes	28 minutes	16 brownies	Mild to medium

INGREDIENTS

1/2 cup (120 g) sourdough discard, cold
1/2 cup (113 g) unsalted butter, cut into pieces
1 cup (170 g) dark chocolate chips or chopped dark chocolate (70% cacao)
1 cup (200 g) granulated sugar
1/2 cup (110 g) packed brown sugar
3 large eggs
1 teaspoon (5 ml) pure vanilla extract

3/4 cup (90 g) all-purpose flour
1/4 cup (25 g) unsweetened cocoa powder
1/2 teaspoon (3 g) fine salt
1/4 teaspoon (1 g) baking powder

INSTRUCTIONS

1. Preheat oven to 350 degrees F (175 degrees C). Line an 8x8-inch baking pan with parchment, leaving an overhang on two sides for easy removal.
2. Melt the butter and chocolate together in a heatproof bowl set over a saucepan of simmering water, stirring until smooth. Alternatively, microwave in 30-second bursts, stirring between each. Remove from heat and let cool for 5 minutes.
3. Whisk both sugars into the warm chocolate mixture. Add the eggs one at a time, whisking well after each. Add the vanilla and sourdough discard and whisk until the batter is smooth and slightly thickened.
4. Sift the flour, cocoa powder, salt, and baking powder over the batter. Fold with a spatula until just combined and no dry streaks remain.
5. Pour into the prepared pan and smooth the top. Bake for 25 to 28 minutes, until the top is set and slightly crackled and a toothpick inserted in the center comes out with moist crumbs (not wet batter).
6. Cool completely in the pan before lifting out and cutting. For the cleanest cuts, refrigerate for 30 minutes after cooling, then cut with a sharp knife wiped clean between cuts.

BAKER'S TIP

Underbaking is deliberate with fudgy brownies. The internal temperature should reach around 200 degrees F when done, but the center will still look slightly underdone through the crackled top. If you wait until a toothpick comes out clean, you have gone too far and will have cakey brownies rather than fudgy ones.

Storage: Room temperature in an airtight container up to 4 days. Refrigerate up to 1 week. These are actually best eaten cold or at room temperature the day after baking. Freeze individually wrapped up to 3 months.

Nutritional Information (per brownie, based on 16 brownies)

Calories	Protein	Carbs	Fat	Fiber	Sodium
235	3 g	33 g	11 g	2 g	110 mg

31 BROWN BUTTER SHORTBREAD

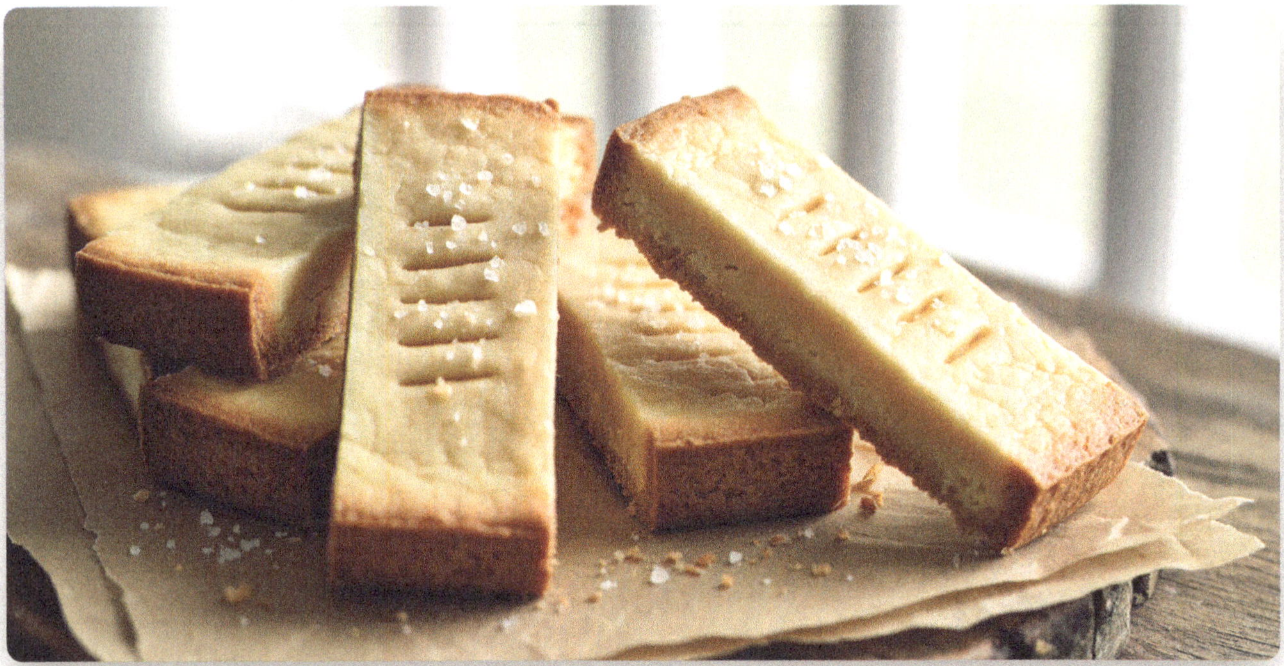

Shortbread is traditionally made with only four ingredients: butter, sugar, flour, and salt. Adding sourdough discard introduces a fifth element that changes the flavor in a way that is subtle and distinctive. The discard's lactic acid interacts with the butter to produce a flavor reminiscent of cultured butter, which makes an already excellent cookie more interesting. Brown butter takes it further. Use mild discard here; the delicate flavor of shortbread cannot absorb assertive tang.

PREP TIME	COOK TIME	YIELD	DISCARD
20 minutes	22 minutes	24 shortbread fingers	Mild only

INGREDIENTS

3/4 cup (170 g) unsalted butter
1/3 cup (80 g) sourdough discard, cold and mild
1/2 cup (60 g) powdered sugar, sifted
1/4 teaspoon (1.5 g) fine salt
1 teaspoon (5 ml) pure vanilla extract
1 3/4 cups (210 g) all-purpose flour
Flaky salt and coarse sugar for topping (optional)

INSTRUCTIONS

1. Brown the butter in a light-colored saucepan over medium heat until the milk solids turn golden and it smells nutty, about 6 minutes. Pour into the bowl of a stand mixer or a large mixing bowl and refrigerate for 30 minutes until it solidifies to a soft, spreadable consistency.
2. Preheat oven to 325 degrees F (165 degrees C). Line a 9x13-inch pan with parchment.
3. Beat the solidified brown butter and powdered sugar together until smooth and slightly fluffy, about 2 minutes. Add the sourdough discard, salt, and vanilla and mix until incorporated.
4. Add the flour and mix on low speed until just combined. The dough will be crumbly at first, then come together as you work it. Do not overmix.
5. Press the dough evenly into the prepared pan in a layer about 1/2 inch thick. Score into fingers (approximately 1x3 inches) with a knife or bench scraper. Prick each piece several times with a fork. Sprinkle with flaky salt and coarse sugar if using.
6. Bake for 20 to 24 minutes until the edges are just beginning to color and the surface looks dry and matte rather than shiny. The shortbread will not brown significantly on top.
7. Remove from the oven and immediately re-cut along the score lines while still warm. Cool completely in the pan before removing.

BAKER'S TIP

Shortbread must be baked low and slow. A higher temperature browns the outside before the interior dries out, producing a cookie with a crunchy shell and a soft, underdone center. At 325 degrees, the heat penetrates evenly and the texture is uniform throughout. Do not be tempted to increase the temperature to speed things up.

Storage: Airtight container at room temperature up to 2 weeks. These keep exceptionally well. Freeze up to 3 months.

Nutritional Information (per finger, based on 24 pieces)

Calories	Protein	Carbs	Fat	Fiber	Sodium
115	2 g	13 g	6 g	0 g	30 mg

PASTRY AND SPECIAL OCCASION

The three recipes in this section are for the moments when you want to make something that looks and tastes genuinely impressive. Each one is more involved than the cookies and bars above, but none of them requires advanced technique. They require attention and patience, which are different things.

32 SOURDOUGH CINNAMON ROLLS

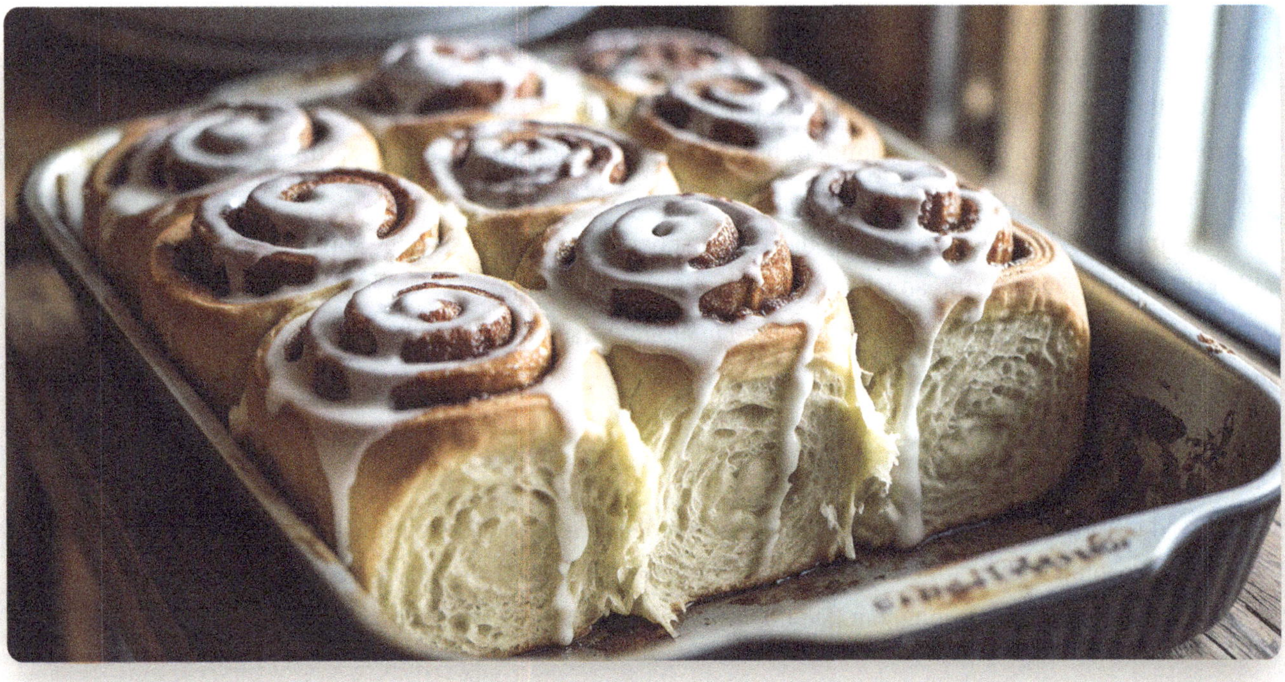

These are enriched dough cinnamon rolls: soft, pull-apart, heavily filled, and finished with a cream cheese glaze. The discard does two things in the dough. It adds flavor that makes the rolls more interesting than plain enriched dough. And its acidity tenderizes the gluten in a way that produces a crumb that is feathery and soft rather than bready and dense. An overnight option is included because the flavor is significantly better after a cold retard in the refrigerator.

PREP TIME	COOK TIME	YIELD	DISCARD
40 min (+ 2 hours rise)	28 minutes	12 rolls	Mild

INGREDIENTS

For the dough:
1/2 cup (120 g) sourdough discard, room temperature
3 cups (360 g) all-purpose flour, plus more for dusting
2 1/4 teaspoons (7 g / 1 packet) instant yeast
1/4 cup (50 g) granulated sugar
1 teaspoon (6 g) fine salt
3/4 cup (180 ml) whole milk, warmed to 110 degrees F
1/4 cup (57 g) unsalted butter, softened
1 large egg
For the filling:
1/2 cup (113 g) unsalted butter, very soft
1 cup (220 g) packed brown sugar
3 tablespoons (18 g) ground cinnamon
1/4 teaspoon (1.5 g) fine salt
For the cream cheese glaze:
4 oz (113 g) cream cheese, softened
1 cup (120 g) powdered sugar, sifted
3 to 4 tablespoons (45 to 60 ml) whole milk
1/2 teaspoon (2.5 ml) pure vanilla extract

INSTRUCTIONS

1. In a large bowl or the bowl of a stand mixer, combine the warm milk, yeast, and sugar. Let sit for 5 minutes until the yeast is foamy, which confirms it is active.
2. Add the sourdough discard, egg, and softened butter to the yeast mixture and mix briefly to combine. Add the flour and salt and knead until a smooth, slightly tacky dough forms, about 8 minutes by machine or 12 minutes by hand. The dough should be soft, elastic, and pull away from the sides of the bowl cleanly.
3. Place the dough in a lightly greased bowl, cover, and let rise at room temperature until doubled in size, 1 to 1.5 hours.
4. While the dough rises, make the filling by combining the soft butter, brown sugar, cinnamon, and salt until smooth.

5. Turn the dough out onto a lightly floured surface and roll into a rectangle approximately 16x12 inches. Spread the filling evenly over the surface, leaving a 1/2-inch border along one of the long edges.
6. Starting from the long edge with filling all the way to the edge, roll the dough tightly into a log. Pinch the seam to seal. Cut into 12 equal rolls with a sharp knife or unflavored dental floss.
7. Place the rolls cut-side up in a greased 9x13-inch pan. Cover and let rise for 45 to 60 minutes until puffed and touching. Alternatively, cover tightly and refrigerate overnight. In the morning, remove from the refrigerator 30 minutes before baking.
8. Preheat oven to 350 degrees F (175 degrees C). Bake for 25 to 28 minutes until the tops are golden and the internal temperature reaches 190 degrees F.
9. While the rolls bake, make the glaze by beating the cream cheese until smooth, then mixing in the powdered sugar, milk, and vanilla until pourable. Spread or drizzle over the hot rolls immediately after baking.

BAKER'S TIP

This recipe uses both yeast and sourdough discard, which might seem redundant. The yeast provides reliable, predictable rise so the rolls are ready in a reasonable time. The discard provides flavor. They are doing different jobs, and both are necessary for the best result.

Storage: Covered at room temperature up to 2 days. Reheat individual rolls in the microwave for 25 seconds. Freeze glazed or unglazed up to 2 months; reheat from frozen in a 300 degrees F oven for 15 minutes covered with foil.

Nutritional Information (per roll, with glaze)

Calories	Protein	Carbs	Fat	Fiber	Sodium
380	7 g	58 g	14 g	2 g	290 mg

33 NO-BAKE CREPE CAKE

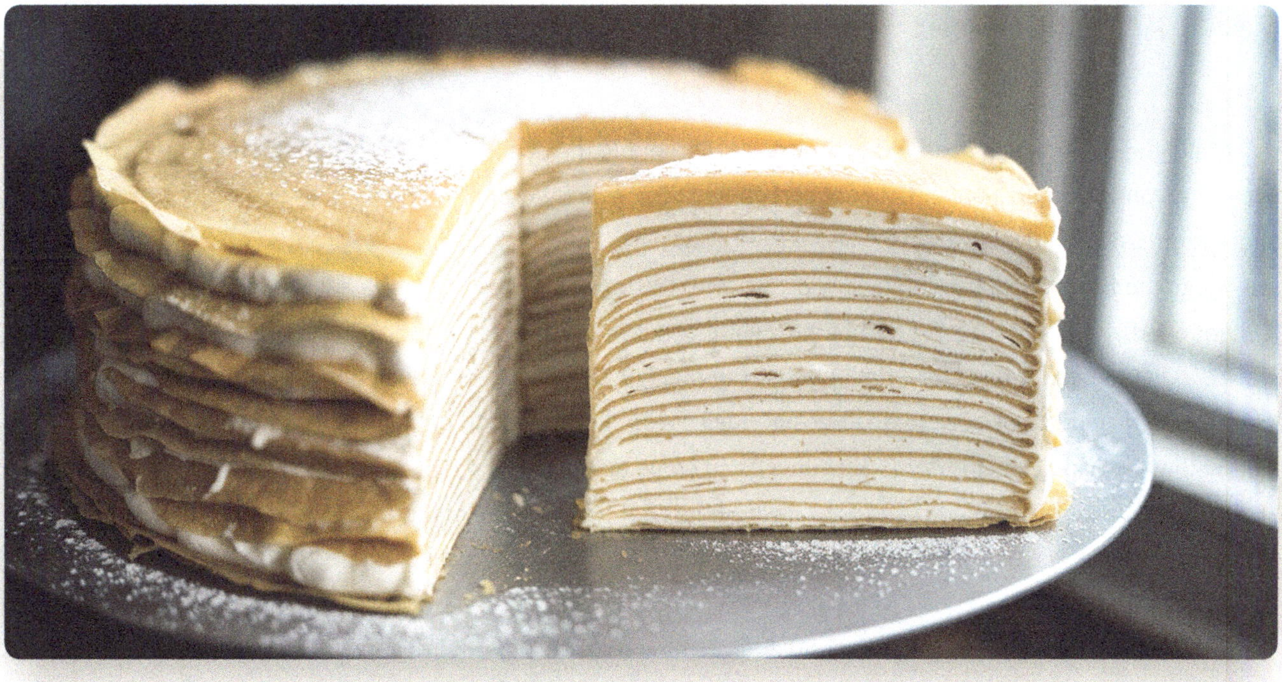

A crepe cake is thirty layers of thin crepes stacked with whipped cream or pastry cream between each layer, sliced like a layer cake to reveal the striped interior. It sounds elaborate but is almost entirely assembly work after the crepes are made. The discard crepe recipe from Chapter 3 (Recipe 11) is the foundation. This is what you make when you want to bring something visually striking to the table without turning on the oven.

PREP TIME 45 minutes	COOK TIME No baking	YIELD One 9-inch cake (10 slices)	DISCARD Mild

INGREDIENTS

For the crepes (makes about 30):

Double batch of the Sourdough Discard Crepe batter from Recipe 11, sweet version

For the whipped cream filling:

2 cups (480 ml) heavy whipping cream, very cold

3 tablespoons (23 g) powdered sugar

1 teaspoon (5 ml) pure vanilla extract

Pinch of fine salt

For finishing:

Powdered sugar for dusting, fresh berries, or thin caramel drizzle

INSTRUCTIONS

1. Make the crepe batter as described in Recipe 11, double the quantities. Rest for 30 minutes, then cook all the crepes and stack on a plate. Let cool completely. You need at least 24 crepes; 28 to 30 produces a taller, more impressive cake.
2. Make the filling: beat the cold heavy cream with the powdered sugar, vanilla, and salt until stiff peaks form. Do not overbeat. Transfer to the refrigerator while you assemble.
3. To assemble: place one crepe flat on a serving plate or cake board. Spread a thin, even layer of whipped cream over the entire surface, going almost to the edges. Place a second crepe on top and press gently. Repeat, alternating crepe and cream, finishing with a plain crepe on top.
4. Refrigerate the assembled cake for at least 2 hours before slicing. This resting time is essential: it allows the layers to set and the cream to firm, which makes clean slicing possible and prevents the cake from sliding when cut.
5. Before serving, dust with powdered sugar and top with fresh berries if desired. Slice with a sharp knife using gentle downward pressure rather than a sawing motion.

BAKER'S TIP

The crepes must be completely cool and the whipped cream must be very stiff before assembly. Warm crepes will melt the cream. Soft cream will make the layers slide. Chill both thoroughly and the assembly will go smoothly.

Storage: Refrigerate assembled, covered loosely, up to 2 days. Do not freeze. Individual crepes (without filling) freeze well for up to 2 months.

Nutritional Information (per slice, based on 10 slices)

Calories	Protein	Carbs	Fat	Fiber	Sodium
285	5 g	22 g	20 g	0 g	95 mg

34 SOURDOUGH DISCARD TART SHELL

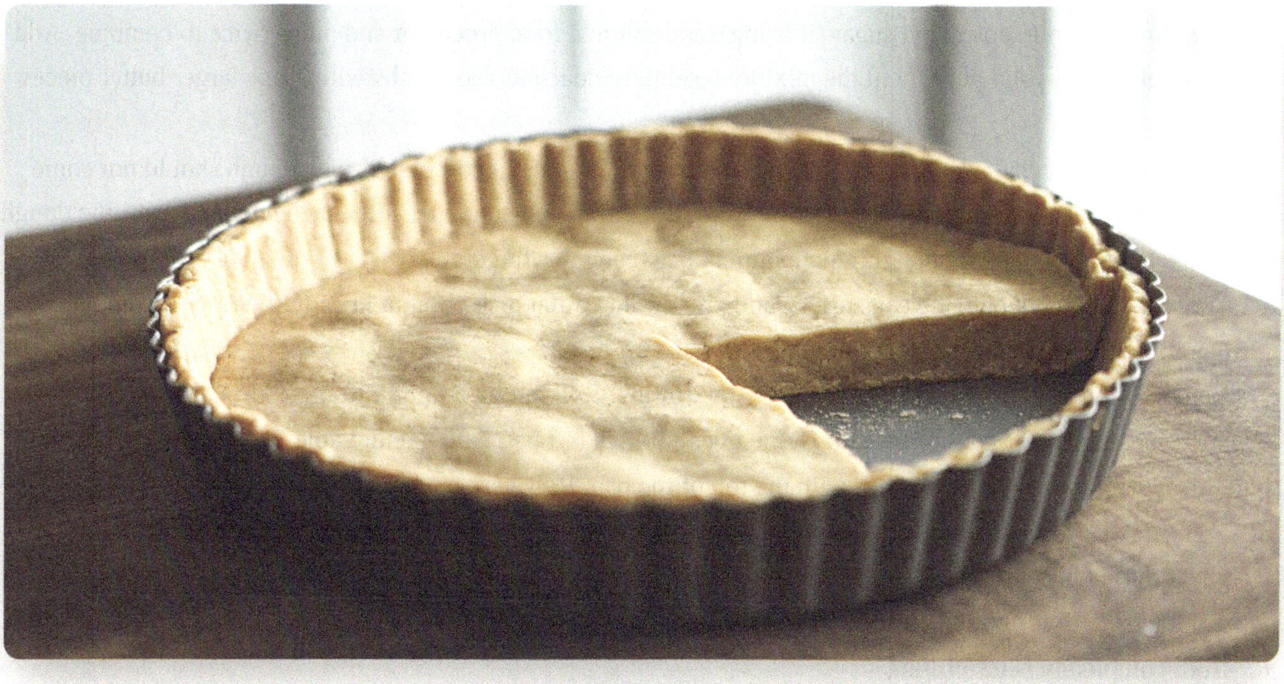

A good tart shell is one of the most versatile things in the baking repertoire: it can be filled with pastry cream and fresh fruit, chocolate ganache, lemon curd, savory custard, or caramelized onions and goat cheese. This shell uses sourdough discard to replace some of the water in a traditional pate sucree (sweet tart pastry), which makes it more tender, more flavorful, and slightly more forgiving to work with. One base recipe, unlimited applications.

PREP TIME **20 min (+ 1 hour chill)**	**COOK TIME** **25 minutes**	**YIELD One** **9-inch tart shell**	**DISCARD** **Mild only**

INGREDIENTS

1 1/4 cups (150 g) all-purpose flour

1/4 cup (30 g) powdered sugar (for sweet shell) OR 1/4 teaspoon salt and no sugar (for savory shell)

1/4 teaspoon (1.5 g) fine salt (both versions)

1/2 cup (113 g) unsalted butter, cold and cut into small cubes

3 tablespoons (45 g) sourdough discard, cold and mild

1 to 2 tablespoons (15 to 30 ml) ice water, added as needed

INSTRUCTIONS

1. Combine the flour, powdered sugar (if using), and salt in a food processor and pulse twice to combine. Add the cold butter cubes and pulse until the mixture resembles coarse breadcrumbs with a few larger butter pieces remaining.
2. Add the sourdough discard and pulse 3 to 4 times until it is just incorporated. The dough should not come together into a ball yet. Add ice water one tablespoon at a time, pulsing once after each addition, until the dough just holds together when you press a small amount between your fingers.
3. Turn the dough out onto a clean surface and press it into a flat disk without kneading. Wrap tightly and refrigerate for at least 1 hour and up to 2 days.
4. Remove from the refrigerator 5 minutes before rolling. Roll out on a lightly floured surface into a circle about 12 inches across and 3 mm thick. Drape over a 9-inch tart pan with a removable bottom and press gently into the edges. Trim any excess flush with the top of the pan. Refrigerate for 20 more minutes.
5. Preheat oven to 375 degrees F (190 degrees C). Line the chilled shell with parchment and fill with pie weights or dried beans. Blind bake for 15 minutes. Remove the weights and parchment and bake for 8 to 10 more minutes until the bottom is fully golden and dry.
6. Cool completely before filling.

BAKER'S TIP

Do not skip the blind bake. A tart shell filled without pre-baking will have a soggy, undercooked bottom. The pie weights prevent the sides from shrinking during the initial bake. If you do not have pie weights, fill with dried beans or rice, which work equally well and can be reused indefinitely for this purpose.

Storage: Baked unfilled shell: room temperature up to 2 days or freeze up to 1 month. Unbaked dough disk: refrigerate up to 2 days or freeze up to 1 month.

Nutritional Information (per slice, based on 10 slices, shell only)

Calories	Protein	Carbs	Fat	Fiber	Sodium
175	3 g	18 g	10 g	1 g	120 mg

CHAPTER 6

Savory Bites

Every chapter in this book so far has leaned toward the morning and the sweet. This chapter corrects that. These eight recipes cover the savory side of what discard can do outside of breakfast: coatings and batters for frying, and baked savory breads that work as snacks, sides, or a light meal with something alongside them.

Discard has two distinct roles in savory cooking. The first is as a batter or coating, where its acidity reacts with the heat of hot oil to produce a crispier, more complex crust than plain flour batter can achieve. The second is as a dough enricher, where it adds flavor and tenderness to baked goods that would otherwise be straightforward but unremarkable.

Both roles are represented in this chapter. The coatings and batters section covers four recipes where discard is the vehicle for crunch. The savory baked section covers four recipes where discard is the background that makes the flavor of the finished bread more interesting than it would be without it.

The acidity in sourdough discard does something in hot oil that buttermilk does in a cold marinade. It begins to break down the surface proteins of whatever you are frying, which creates a crust that adheres more cleanly and stays crispy longer after it comes out of the oil.

A note on frying: three of the four coating and batter recipes involve hot oil. None of them require a deep fryer. A heavy-bottomed pot with 2 to 3 inches of oil, a thermometer, and a slotted spoon are all the equipment you need. Temperature control is the only technique that matters. Oil that is too cool produces greasy, soggy coatings. Oil that is too hot burns the outside before the inside cooks. Every recipe gives a specific temperature and explains how to maintain it.

COATINGS AND BATTERS

35 DISCARD FRIED CHICKEN

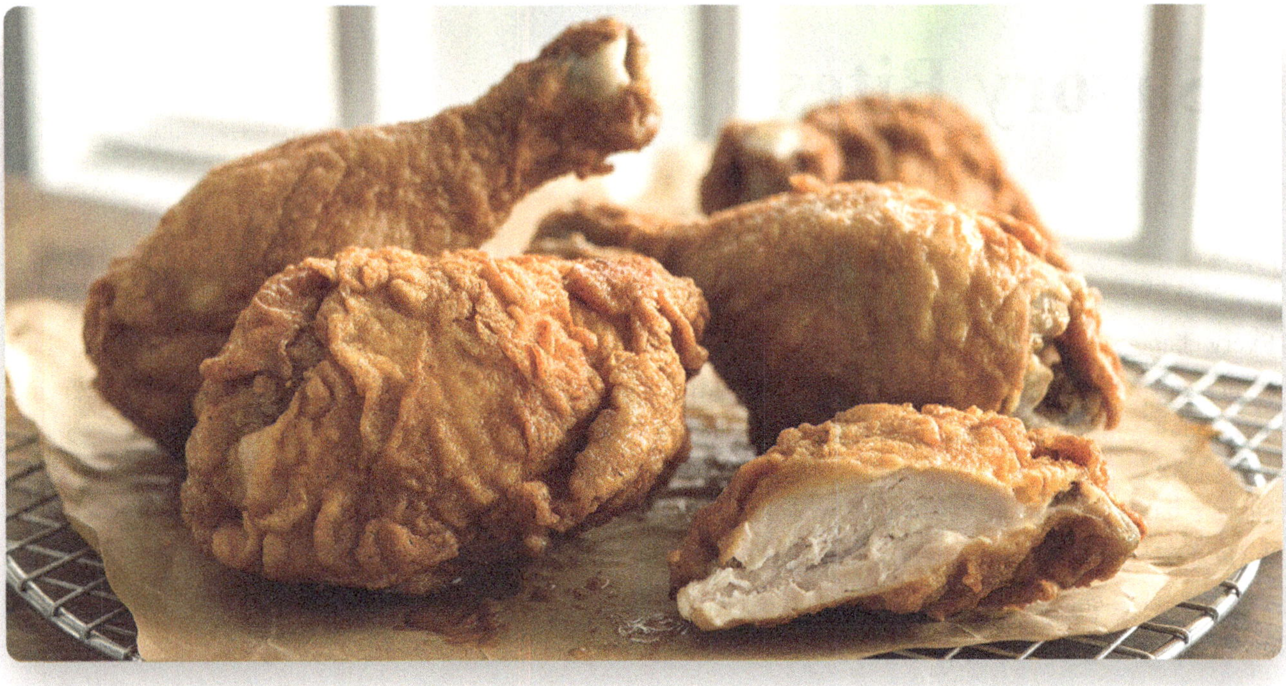

Fried chicken coated in sourdough discard batter has a distinctly different crust than buttermilk fried chicken. The crust is thinner and crisper rather than thick and craggy, and it adheres to the chicken more completely during frying, which means less coating falling off in the oil and more on the chicken. The discard also begins a very gentle tenderizing process on the chicken surface during the marinating time, producing a juicier result than an unfermented coating.

PREP TIME	COOK TIME	YIELD	DISCARD
20 min (+ 4 hour marinate)	25 minutes	4 servings	Medium to tangy

INGREDIENTS

For the marinade:

1/2 cup (120 g) sourdough discard

1/2 cup (120 ml) whole milk

1 teaspoon (6 g) fine salt

1/2 teaspoon (1 g) black pepper

1/2 teaspoon (1 g) garlic powder

1/2 teaspoon (1 g) smoked paprika

2 lbs (900 g) bone-in, skin-on chicken pieces (thighs and drumsticks work best)

For the coating:

1 1/2 cups (180 g) all-purpose flour

1 teaspoon (6 g) fine salt

1 teaspoon (2 g) black pepper

1 teaspoon (2 g) garlic powder

1 teaspoon (2 g) smoked paprika

1/2 teaspoon (1 g) cayenne pepper (optional)

Neutral oil for frying (vegetable, canola, or peanut)

INSTRUCTIONS

1. Combine the discard, milk, salt, pepper, garlic powder, and smoked paprika in a large bowl or zip-lock bag. Add the chicken pieces, turning to coat completely. Refrigerate for at least 4 hours and up to 24 hours. Longer marinating produces more flavor and more tender chicken.
2. When ready to fry, remove the chicken from the refrigerator 30 minutes before cooking to take the chill off. Cold chicken dropped into hot oil lowers the oil temperature dramatically and produces uneven cooking.
3. Combine all the coating ingredients in a shallow dish and mix well. Remove each piece of chicken from the marinade, letting the excess drip off, and dredge thoroughly in the seasoned flour. Press the flour into the surface firmly. Let the coated chicken rest on a wire rack for 10 minutes before frying. This resting time allows the coating to adhere and become slightly tacky, which reduces shedding in the oil.
4. Pour oil into a heavy-bottomed pot or Dutch oven to a depth of 3 inches. Heat to 325 degrees F (165 degrees C). Use a thermometer. This temperature is lower than many fried chicken recipes because bone-in pieces need time for the heat to penetrate to the bone without burning the outside.
5. Fry 2 to 3 pieces at a time, maintaining the oil temperature between 300 and 325 degrees F. Do not crowd the pot. Fry thighs and drumsticks for 12 to 14 minutes total, turning occasionally, until deep golden brown and the internal temperature reaches 165 degrees F.
6. Transfer to a wire rack set over a sheet pan to drain. Do not use paper towels as a resting surface as they trap steam and soften the crust. Season immediately with a light pinch of salt.

BAKER'S TIP

The single most important variable in frying is maintaining consistent oil temperature. Every piece of cold chicken you add drops the temperature. Add the chicken slowly, wait for the oil to recover between additions, and never cook more than 3 pieces at a time in a standard pot. A clip-on thermometer makes this easy to monitor continuously.

Storage: Best eaten immediately. Leftovers can be refrigerated up to 3 days and reheated in a 375 degree F oven for 15 minutes on a wire rack, which restores some crispness. Do not reheat in a microwave as it makes the coating soggy.

Nutritional Information (per serving, skin-on, fried in oil)

Calories	Protein	Carbs	Fat	Fiber	Sodium
490	38 g	32 g	22 g	1 g	680 mg

36 FISH AND CHIP BATTER

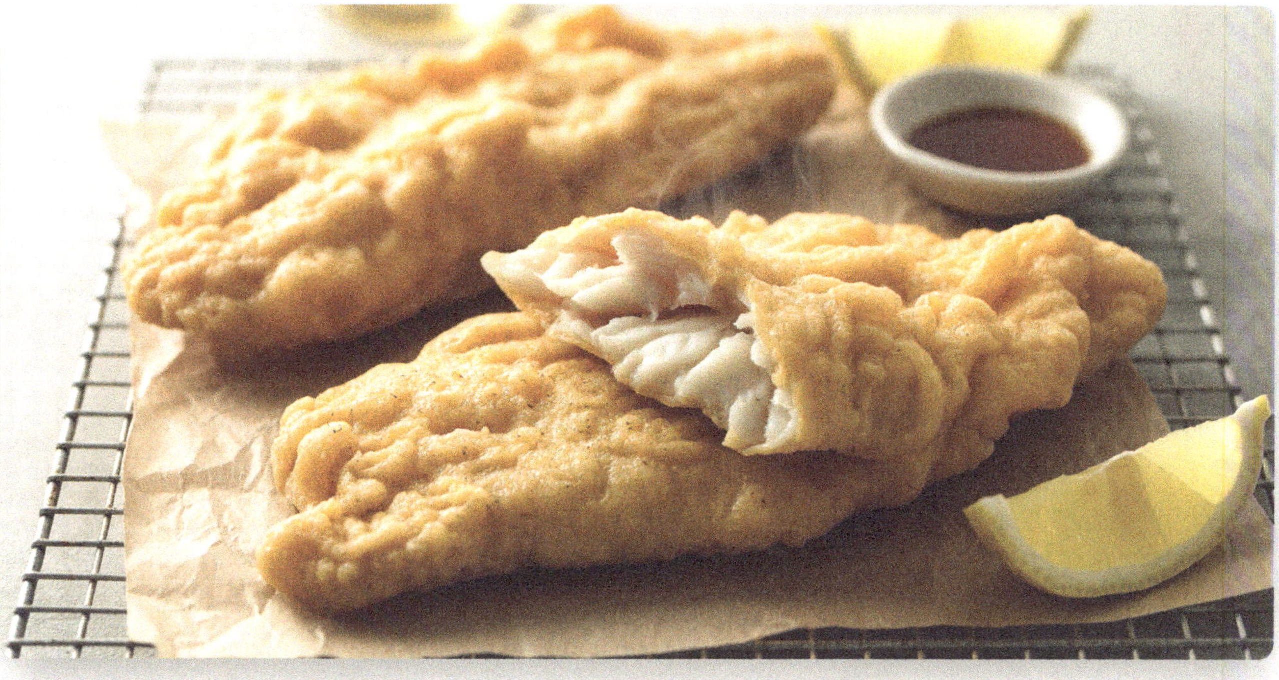

This is a pub-style batter: light, crispy, and slightly shattering when bitten. Traditional beer batter uses carbonation to lighten the crust. Sourdough discard achieves the same effect through a different mechanism. The yeast activity in the discard produces small amounts of carbon dioxide when it hits the hot oil, creating bubbles in the batter that make it airy and delicate rather than dense and doughy. The result is a crust with genuine crunch that holds for 10 to 15 minutes after frying.

PREP TIME	COOK TIME	YIELD	DISCARD
15 minutes	20 minutes	4 servings	Medium

INGREDIENTS

For the batter:
3/4 cup (180 g) sourdough discard, cold
3/4 cup (90 g) all-purpose flour
1/4 cup (30 g) rice flour or cornstarch (adds crispness)
1 teaspoon (4 g) baking powder
1/2 teaspoon (3 g) fine salt
1/4 teaspoon (0.5 g) white pepper

1/2 cup (120 ml) cold sparkling water or cold plain water

For the fish:

5 lbs (680 g) firm white fish fillets (cod, haddock, or halibut), cut into pieces about 4 inches long

Fine salt and pepper

1/4 cup (30 g) all-purpose flour for dusting

Neutral oil for frying

INSTRUCTIONS

1. Pat the fish fillets completely dry with paper towels. Season lightly with salt and pepper. Dredge each piece lightly in plain flour, shaking off the excess. The flour dusting gives the batter something to grip.
2. Make the batter just before frying: whisk together the discard, flour, rice flour, baking powder, salt, and white pepper. Add the cold water and whisk until just smooth. A few small lumps are acceptable. Do not overmix and do not let the batter sit for more than 5 minutes before using.
3. Heat 3 inches of oil in a heavy pot to 375 degrees F (190 degrees C). This higher temperature is appropriate for fish, which cooks quickly and needs rapid crust formation to stay juicy inside.
4. Dip each piece of flour-dusted fish into the batter, letting the excess drip off, and lower gently into the hot oil. Fry 2 pieces at a time for 4 to 5 minutes, turning once, until deep golden and crispy. Internal temperature should reach 145 degrees F.
5. Drain on a wire rack and serve immediately with malt vinegar, tartar sauce, or lemon wedges.

BAKER'S TIP

Cold batter and hot oil are the two keys to a light, crispy fish crust. Warm batter absorbs more oil and produces a heavier result. Keep the batter in the refrigerator between batches if you are cooking multiple rounds. If the batter thickens as it sits, thin it with a tablespoon of cold water.

Storage: Fried fish is best eaten immediately and does not keep well. The batter can be made up to 30 minutes ahead and kept refrigerated.

Nutritional Information (per serving)

Calories	Protein	Carbs	Fat	Fiber	Sodium
385	32 g	28 g	16 g	1 g	520 mg

37 TEMPURA VEGETABLE FRITTERS

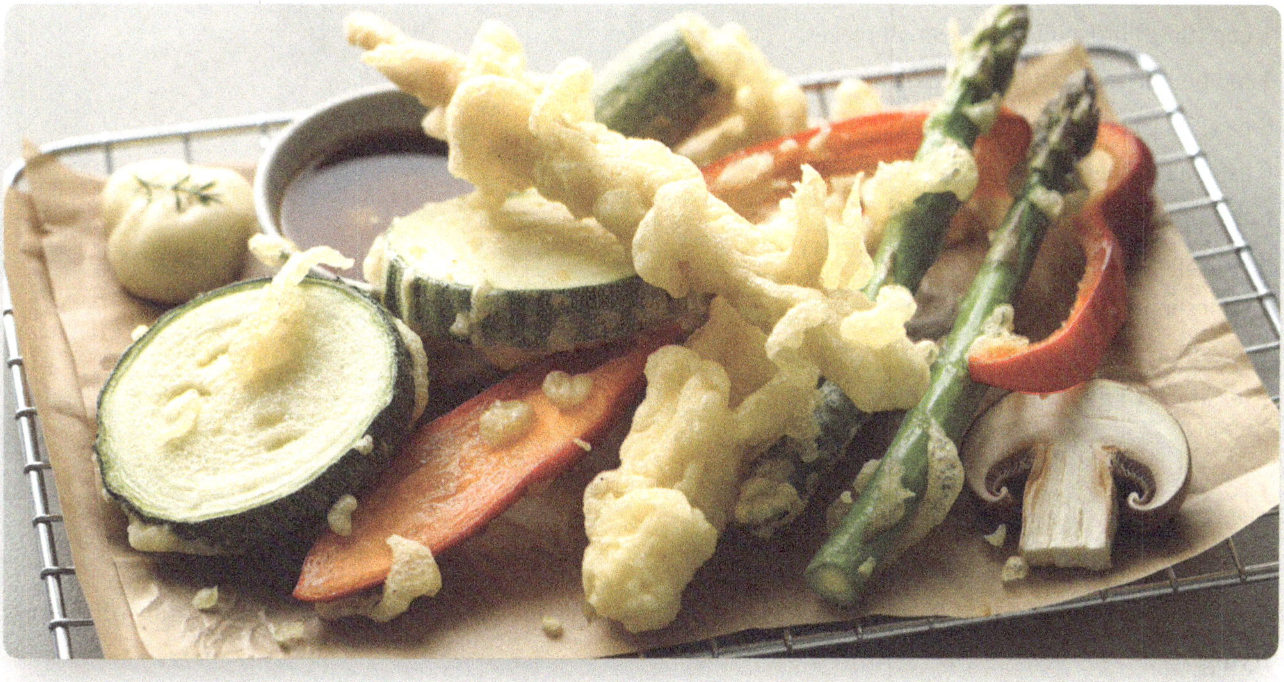

Traditional tempura uses ice-cold water and minimal mixing to produce an extremely light, delicate batter that barely coats the vegetable. Sourdough discard added to this formula contributes flavor and a slightly more substantial coating without sacrificing the lightness that makes tempura different from ordinary fried vegetables. This version works with almost any vegetable: the list below is a starting point.

PREP TIME 15 minutes	COOK TIME 20 minutes	YIELD 4 servings	DISCARD Mild to medium

INGREDIENTS

For the batter:

1/3 cup (80 g) sourdough discard, cold

1 cup (120 g) all-purpose flour

2 tablespoons (16 g) cornstarch

1/2 teaspoon (3 g) fine salt

3/4 cup (180 ml) ice-cold sparkling water (flat water also works but sparkling is better)

1 large egg yolk

Suggested vegetables (use any combination):
1 medium zucchini, sliced into 1/4-inch rounds
1 medium sweet potato, peeled and sliced into 1/8-inch rounds
1 cup (90 g) broccoli florets, small pieces
1 red bell pepper, cut into strips
8 oz (225 g) cremini mushrooms, halved
8 asparagus spears, trimmed and cut in half
For dipping:
3 tablespoons (45 ml) soy sauce
1 tablespoon (15 ml) rice vinegar
1 teaspoon (5 ml) sesame oil
1 teaspoon (4 g) grated fresh ginger

INSTRUCTIONS

1. Prepare all vegetables and pat completely dry. Any surface moisture will cause the batter to slide off during frying.
2. Make the dipping sauce by combining the soy sauce, rice vinegar, sesame oil, and ginger. Set aside.
3. Heat 3 inches of oil to 350 degrees F (175 degrees C) in a heavy pot.
4. Make the batter immediately before frying: whisk together the flour, cornstarch, and salt in a medium bowl. In a separate small bowl, whisk the discard, ice water, and egg yolk together briefly. Pour the wet ingredients into the dry and stir with chopsticks or a fork just 4 to 5 times. The batter should be lumpy and look almost unmixed. This deliberate undermixing is what keeps tempura light.
5. Working in small batches, dip vegetables into the batter, let the excess drip off, and lower into the hot oil. Fry for 2 to 3 minutes until the batter is set and just beginning to color. Tempura should be pale golden, not deep brown.
6. Drain on a wire rack. Serve immediately with the dipping sauce.

BAKER'S TIP

Tempura batter deteriorates quickly. Make it in small amounts and use it fast. If you are frying a large quantity of vegetables, make two half-batches of batter rather than one large batch, keeping the second half refrigerated until needed. Warm, well-mixed batter produces dense, greasy tempura.

Storage: Eat immediately. Tempura does not hold well and should not be reheated.

Nutritional Information (per serving, mixed vegetables)

Calories	Protein	Carbs	Fat	Fiber	Sodium
260	7 g	38 g	9 g	3 g	520 mg

38 DISCARD ONION RINGS

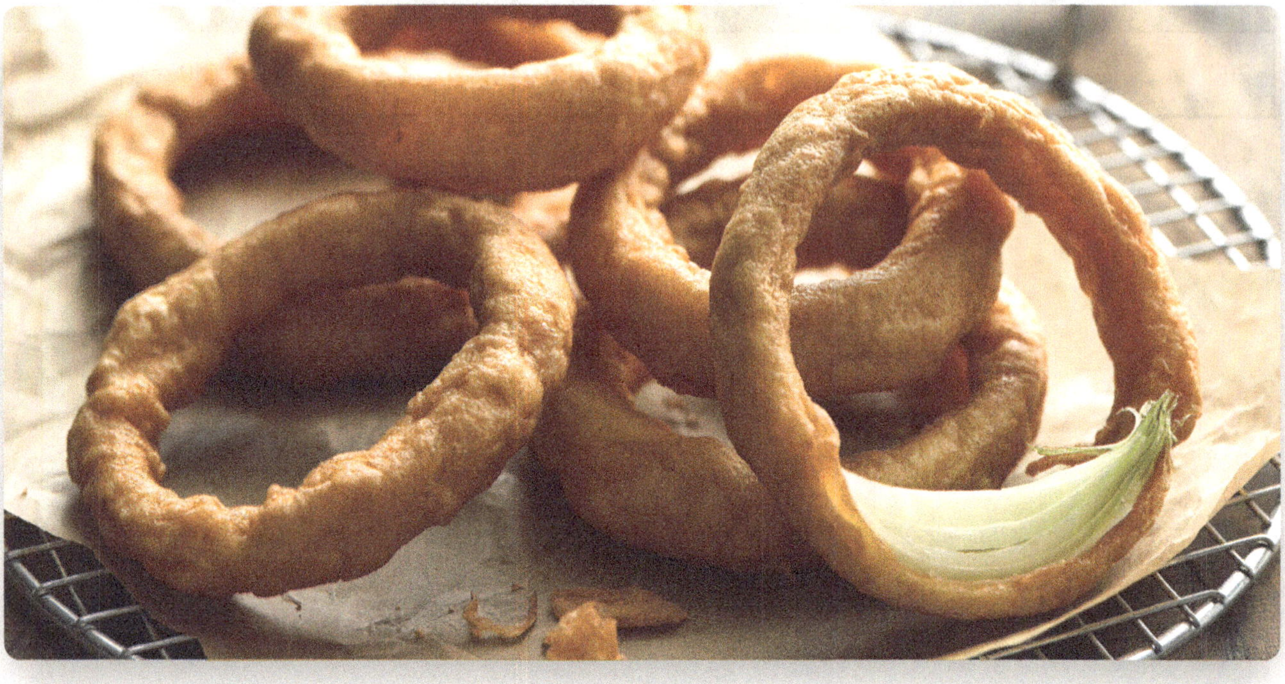

These are thick-cut, substantial onion rings with a batter that clings completely and stays crispy for longer than most onion ring recipes. The discard adds a slight tang to the coating that plays well against the sweetness of a cooked onion. Sweet onions (Vidalia or Walla Walla) work best here because their lower sulfur content means they cook through completely in the frying time without becoming sharp.

PREP TIME	COOK TIME	YIELD	DISCARD
15 minutes	20 minutes	4 servings	Medium

INGREDIENTS

2 large sweet onions, peeled and cut into 1/2-inch rings
1/2 cup (120 g) sourdough discard, cold
1 cup (120 g) all-purpose flour, plus 1/4 cup (30 g) for dusting
1/4 cup (30 g) cornstarch
1 teaspoon (4 g) baking powder
1 teaspoon (6 g) fine salt, plus more for finishing
1/2 teaspoon (1 g) black pepper

1/2 teaspoon (1 g) garlic powder
1/2 teaspoon (1 g) smoked paprika
3/4 cup (180 ml) cold sparkling water
Neutral oil for frying

INSTRUCTIONS

1. Separate the onion rings and place them on a sheet pan. Dust lightly all over with the 1/4 cup of plain flour. The flour dusting is what allows the batter to adhere to the onion's slick surface.
2. Make the batter: whisk together the 1 cup flour, cornstarch, baking powder, salt, pepper, garlic powder, and paprika. Add the discard and cold sparkling water and whisk until just smooth.
3. Heat 3 inches of oil to 375 degrees F (190 degrees C).
4. Working in batches of 4 to 6 rings, dip each floured ring into the batter, let the excess drip off, and lay gently into the hot oil. Do not overlap rings in the oil. Fry for 3 to 4 minutes, turning once, until deep golden all over.
5. Transfer to a wire rack and season immediately with a pinch of fine salt. Serve within 10 minutes.

BAKER'S TIP

The most common onion ring mistake is using yellow onions rather than sweet onions. Yellow onions are sharper and take longer to cook through, which means by the time the interior is soft the exterior batter is often overdone. Sweet onions cook through in the same time it takes the batter to crisp, producing a ring that is soft and sweet inside with a crunchy exterior.

Storage: Best eaten immediately. The batter softens within 20 minutes and does not reheat successfully.

Nutritional Information (per serving)

Calories	Protein	Carbs	Fat	Fiber	Sodium
320	6 g	42 g	14 g	2 g	580 mg

SAVORY BAKED

These four recipes use discard as a dough enricher rather than as a coating. In each case the discard is doing the same job: adding flavor to a dough that would be competent but forgettable without it. The difference between a pretzel made with discard and one made without is not dramatic. It is the kind of improvement you notice on the second bite and can no longer attribute to any single ingredient.

39 SOFT PRETZELS

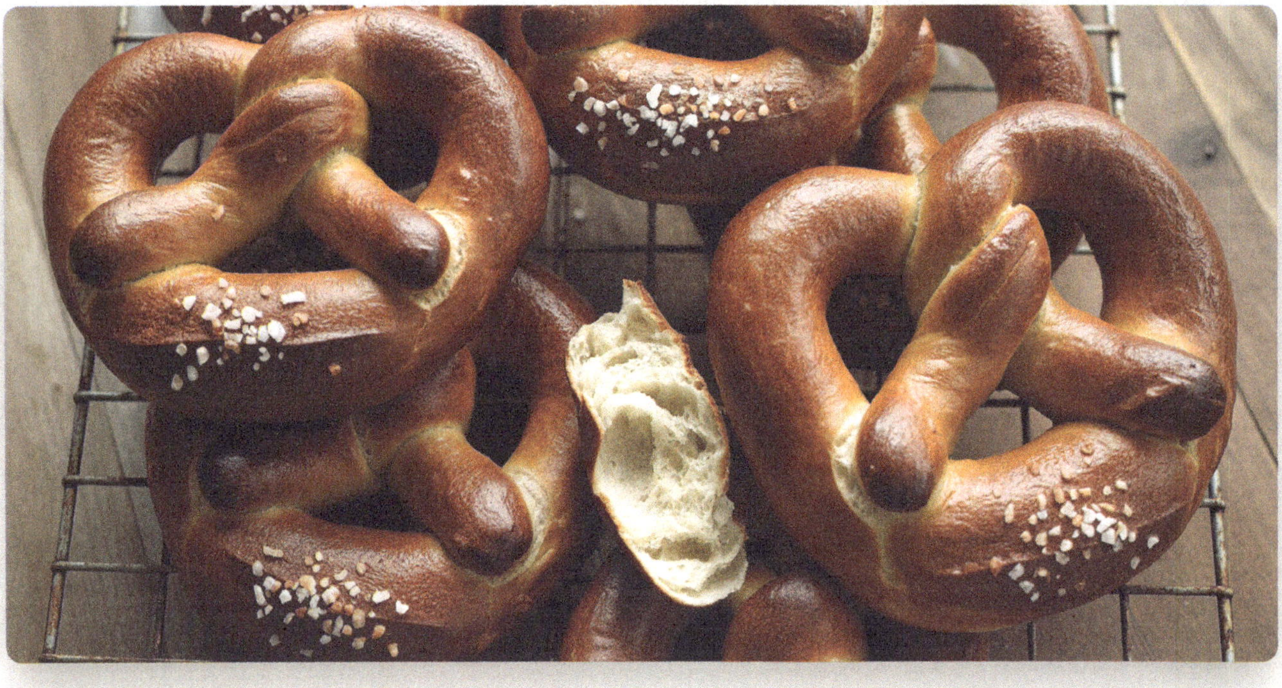

Traditional soft pretzels are dipped in lye solution before baking, which produces the characteristic dark mahogany crust and distinctive chewy texture. This recipe uses a baked baking soda bath instead, which is safer for home kitchens and produces a very similar result. Sourdough discard in the dough adds the subtle tang that makes a pretzel taste like a pretzel rather than a shaped bread roll.

PREP TIME	COOK TIME	YIELD	DISCARD
30 min (+ 1 hour rise)	15 minutes	8 pretzels	Medium to tangy

INGREDIENTS

For the dough:
1/2 cup (120 g) sourdough discard, room temperature
2 1/4 teaspoons (7 g / 1 packet) instant yeast
1 cup (240 ml) warm water (110 degrees F)
1 tablespoon (12 g) granulated sugar
3 cups (360 g) all-purpose flour, plus more for kneading
1 1/2 teaspoons (9 g) fine salt
2 tablespoons (28 g) unsalted butter, softened
For the baking soda bath:
8 cups (1.9 liters) water
1/3 cup (75 g) baking soda
For finishing:
1 egg yolk beaten with 1 tablespoon water (egg wash)
Coarse pretzel salt or flaky salt

INSTRUCTIONS

1. Combine the warm water, yeast, and sugar in a large bowl. Let stand 5 minutes until foamy.
2. Add the sourdough discard, flour, salt, and softened butter. Mix until a shaggy dough forms, then knead on a lightly floured surface for 8 to 10 minutes until the dough is smooth, elastic, and slightly tacky. It should spring back slowly when you press a finger into it.
3. Place in a lightly greased bowl, cover, and let rise at room temperature for 1 hour until doubled.
4. Preheat oven to 450 degrees F (230 degrees C). Line two baking sheets with parchment and grease the parchment.
5. Bring the water to a boil in a wide pot. Carefully add the baking soda. It will foam vigorously. Stir to dissolve and reduce to a gentle simmer.
6. Divide the dough into 8 equal pieces. Roll each piece into a rope about 22 inches long. Shape into a pretzel: form a U shape, cross the ends twice, then fold them down and press them to the bottom of the U.
7. Boil each pretzel in the baking soda bath for 30 seconds, turning once. Remove with a slotted spatula and place on the prepared baking sheets. Brush with egg wash and sprinkle generously with coarse salt.

8. Bake for 13 to 15 minutes until deep mahogany brown. Cool on a wire rack for 5 minutes before eating.

BAKER'S TIP

The baking soda bath is what makes a pretzel a pretzel rather than a bread roll. The alkaline solution raises the pH of the dough surface, which causes rapid browning through a different chemical reaction than ordinary caramelization. Do not skip this step, and do not substitute plain water. The baking soda bath is responsible for the crust, the color, and a significant portion of the flavor.

Storage: Best eaten the day they are made. Store in a paper bag at room temperature up to 1 day. Reheat in a 350 degree F oven for 5 minutes to restore the crust. Freeze baked pretzels up to 1 month; reheat from frozen at 375 degrees F for 12 minutes.

Nutritional Information (per pretzel, with salt)

Calories	Protein	Carbs	Fat	Fiber	Sodium
265	7 g	47 g	5 g	2 g	1180 mg

40 BREADSTICKS

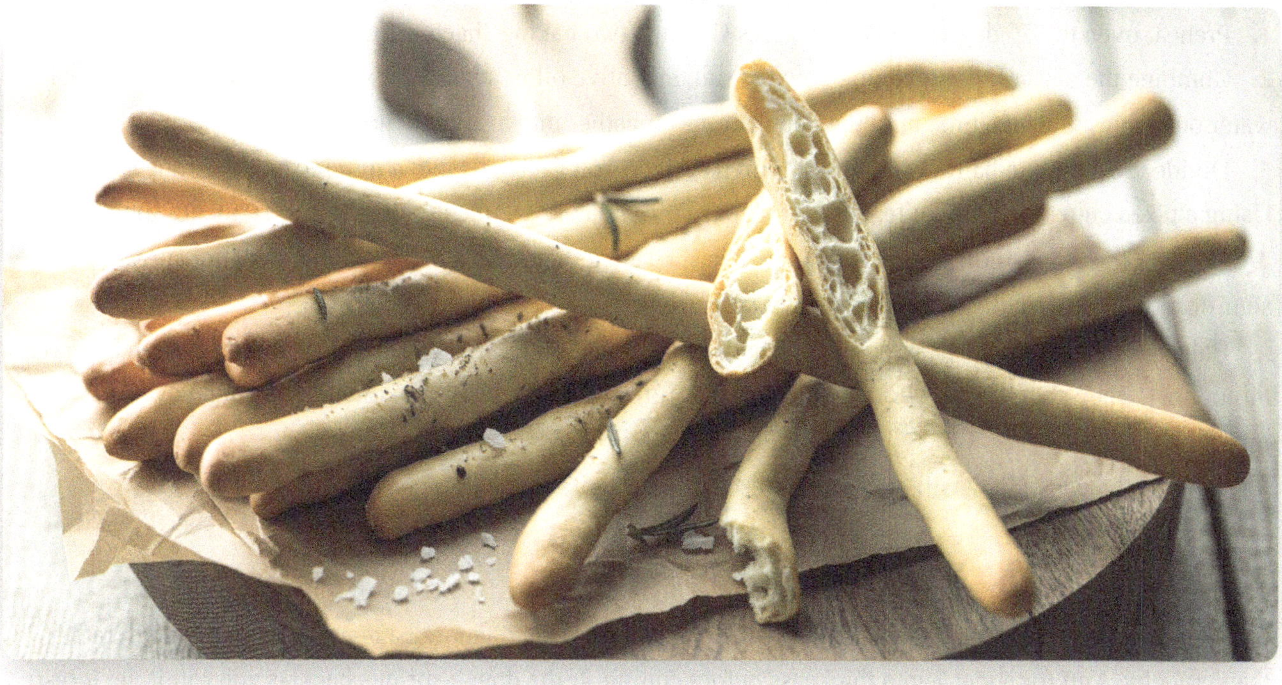

These are thin, crunchy breadsticks in the Italian grissini style, not the soft, doughy variety. They go from bowl to oven in 30 minutes with no rise time required, and they are the thing to make when you want something to put on the table immediately for guests. The discard adds enough flavor that these do not need much help: olive oil, flaky salt, and a light scattering of rosemary is all they require.

PREP TIME	COOK TIME	YIELD	DISCARD
20 minutes	18 minutes	24 breadsticks	Medium

INGREDIENTS

1/2 cup (120 g) sourdough discard, cold
1 1/4 cups (150 g) all-purpose flour
1/2 teaspoon (2 g) baking powder
1/2 teaspoon (3 g) fine salt
3 tablespoons (45 ml) olive oil, plus more for brushing
2 to 3 tablespoons (30 to 45 ml) cold water
Flaky salt, dried rosemary, sesame seeds, or black pepper for topping

INSTRUCTIONS

1. Preheat oven to 375 degrees F (190 degrees C). Line two baking sheets with parchment.
2. Combine the discard, flour, baking powder, salt, and olive oil in a bowl. Mix until crumbly, then add cold water one tablespoon at a time until the dough comes together into a smooth, non-sticky ball.
3. Divide the dough in half. On a lightly floured surface, roll each half into a thin rectangle, about 10x8 inches. Using a pizza cutter or sharp knife, cut into strips approximately 1/2 inch wide and 8 to 10 inches long.
4. Transfer the strips to the prepared baking sheets, spacing them 1/2 inch apart. They will not spread significantly. Brush lightly with olive oil and sprinkle with your chosen toppings.
5. Bake for 16 to 18 minutes, rotating pans halfway through, until the breadsticks are evenly golden and crispy throughout. They should snap cleanly when broken. If the centers are still flexible, return to the oven for 3 more minutes.
6. Cool on the pans. They will crisp further as they cool.

BAKER'S TIP

Roll the dough as thin as you can manage. Thick breadsticks take longer to bake and tend to be tough rather than crunchy. Aim for about 3 mm thickness before cutting. If the dough springs back as you roll it, let it rest for 3 minutes and try again.

Storage: Airtight container at room temperature up to 5 days. These keep well and crisp stays good. Do not refrigerate. If they soften, return to a 300 degree F oven for 5 minutes.

Nutritional Information (per breadstick, plain)

Calories	Protein	Carbs	Fat	Fiber	Sodium
55	1 g	8 g	2 g	0 g	65 mg

41 HAM AND GRUYERE SAVORY SCONES

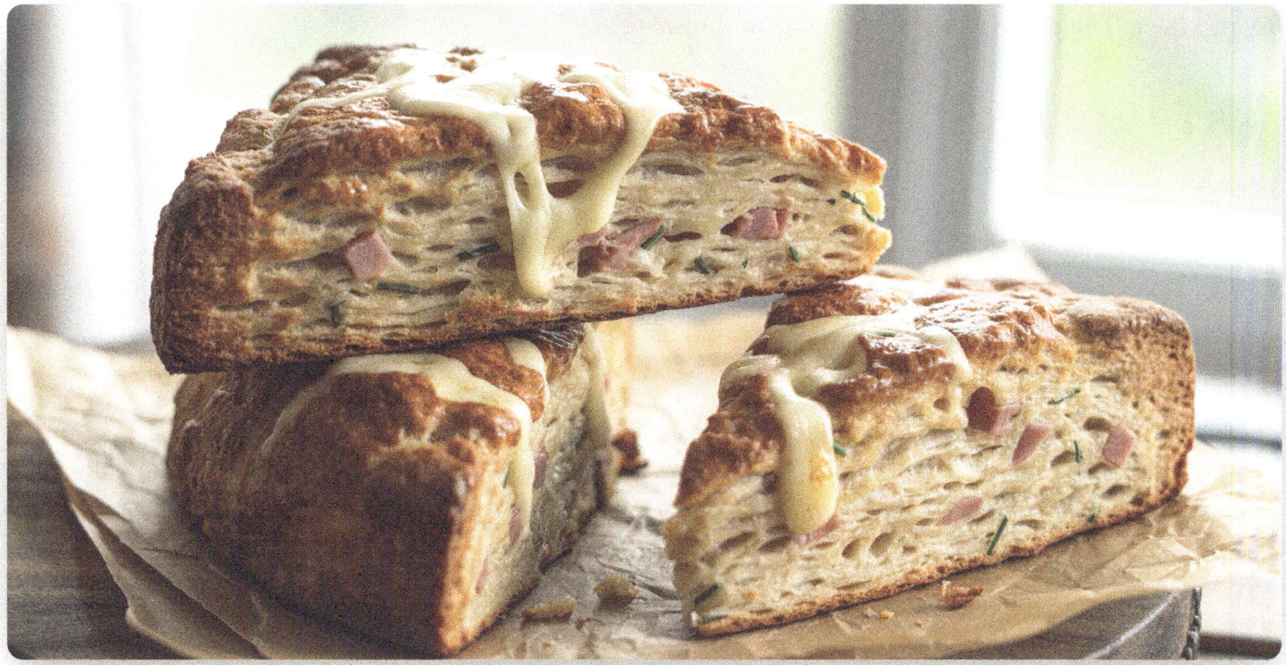

These are substantial, savory scones built on the same lamination technique as the biscuits in Chapter 3. The discard's tang contrasts with the saltiness of the ham and the nuttiness of the gruyere in a way that makes each component taste more defined. They work as a standalone breakfast, a lunch alongside soup, or a snack. The cheese is not optional. It is doing structural as well as flavor work in the dough.

PREP TIME	COOK TIME	YIELD	DISCARD
20 minutes	20 minutes	8 scones	Medium

INGREDIENTS

2 cups (240 g) all-purpose flour
1 tablespoon (12 g) baking powder
1/2 teaspoon (3 g) fine salt
1/4 teaspoon (0.5 g) black pepper
1/4 teaspoon (0.5 g) dry mustard powder
1/2 cup (113 g) unsalted butter, very cold, grated
3/4 cup (85 g) gruyere cheese, shredded (or substitute sharp cheddar)

3/4 cup (110 g) cooked ham, finely diced
2 tablespoons (8 g) fresh chives or scallions, finely sliced
1/2 cup (120 g) sourdough discard, cold
1/4 cup (60 ml) cold heavy cream, plus more for brushing

INSTRUCTIONS

1. Preheat oven to 400 degrees F (205 degrees C). Line a baking sheet with parchment.
2. In a large bowl, whisk together the flour, baking powder, salt, pepper, and mustard powder. Add the grated cold butter and toss until each piece is coated with flour. You should have visible butter shreds throughout, similar to the biscuit dough in Chapter 3.
3. Add the shredded gruyere, diced ham, and chives. Toss to distribute evenly.
4. In a small bowl, stir together the sourdough discard and cold heavy cream. Pour over the flour mixture and fold with a spatula until just combined. The dough will be rough and shaggy. Turn it out onto a lightly floured surface and press together into a disk about 1 inch thick.
5. Cut the disk into 8 wedges like a pie. Transfer to the prepared baking sheet, spacing them 2 inches apart. Brush the tops lightly with cream.
6. Bake for 18 to 20 minutes until the tops are deep golden and the cheese is bubbling at the edges. Cool for 5 minutes on the sheet before serving.

BAKER'S TIP

Do not cut the ham into large chunks. Fine dicing distributes the ham evenly through every bite and prevents the scone from cracking along large inclusions during baking. The same principle applies to the cheese: shredded distributes better than cubed and melts more evenly into the dough.

Storage: Room temperature in an airtight container up to 2 days. Refrigerate up to 4 days. Reheat in a 350 degree F oven for 8 minutes to restore the crust. Freeze up to 2 months; reheat from frozen at 375 degrees F for 15 minutes.

Nutritional Information (per scone)

Calories	Protein	Carbs	Fat	Fiber	Sodium
340	11 g	28 g	20 g	1 g	530 mg

42 SHEET PAN FOCACCIA

This is the most relaxed bread recipe in the book. The dough requires no shaping, almost no kneading, and an extended refrigerator rest that does most of the flavor development work for you. The result is a thick, dimpled, olive oil-soaked focaccia with a crispy bottom and a pillowy interior. The discard amplifies the yeast's flavor contribution and produces a bread that tastes like it came from a good bakery rather than a home kitchen. The topping suggestions below are minimal and right. Focaccia does not need much on top.

PREP TIME 20 min (+ overnight rest)	COOK TIME 25 minutes	YIELD One 18 x 13-inch pan (12 pieces)	DISCARD Medium to tangy

INGREDIENTS

For the dough:
1/2 cup (120 g) sourdough discard, cold
2 1/4 teaspoons (7 g / 1 packet) instant yeast
1 3/4 cups (420 ml) warm water (100 degrees F)
1 tablespoon (12 g) granulated sugar
4 cups (480 g) all-purpose flour
1 1/2 teaspoons (9 g) fine salt
3 tablespoons (45 ml) olive oil, plus more for the pan
For the topping:
1/4 cup (60 ml) good olive oil
Flaky sea salt
Choose one or two: fresh rosemary sprigs, halved cherry tomatoes, thin-sliced red onion, sliced Castelvetrano olives, or roasted garlic cloves

INSTRUCTIONS

1. In a large bowl, combine the warm water, yeast, and sugar. Let stand 5 minutes until foamy. Add the sourdough discard and olive oil and stir briefly.
2. Add the flour and salt and mix with a wooden spoon or your hands until a shaggy, sticky dough forms. Do not knead. Cover the bowl tightly with plastic wrap and refrigerate for 8 to 18 hours. The long cold fermentation is where the flavor develops.

3. When ready to bake, generously coat an 18x13-inch rimmed baking sheet (half sheet pan) with olive oil. A generous pour, about 3 tablespoons, is not excessive here. The oil is what creates the crispy bottom. Pour the cold dough into the oiled pan.
4. With oiled fingertips, gently stretch the dough toward the edges of the pan. It will resist and spring back. Let it rest for 15 minutes, then stretch again. Repeat once more if needed. Eventually it will relax enough to fill the pan. Cover loosely and let rise at room temperature for 1.5 to 2 hours until visibly puffy.
5. Preheat oven to 450 degrees F (230 degrees C). Drizzle the remaining olive oil over the dough surface. With oiled fingertips, press dimples all over the dough, pressing firmly all the way to the bottom of the pan. Add your chosen toppings, pressing them gently in. Sprinkle generously with flaky salt.
6. Bake for 22 to 26 minutes until the top is deep golden and the edges are pulling away from the sides of the pan. The bottom should be audibly crispy when you lift a corner with a spatula. Cool in the pan for 10 minutes before cutting.

BAKER'S TIP

Do not skip the olive oil on the pan. It is not there to prevent sticking only. It crisps the bottom of the focaccia by essentially frying it against the metal as it bakes. A focaccia bottom that is merely oiled rather than generously oiled will be soft rather than crispy. Use a heavy hand with the oil and do not substitute cooking spray.

Storage: Room temperature covered with a towel up to 2 days. Reheat slices in a hot skillet or 400 degree F oven for 5 minutes to restore the crust. Freeze in individual pieces up to 1 month.

Nutritional Information (per piece, based on 12 pieces, plain)

Calories	Protein	Carbs	Fat	Fiber	Sodium
265	6 g	38 g	10 g	2 g	390 mg

CHAPTER 7

One Batter, Many Ways

Every recipe in this book so far has been a standalone thing: a specific outcome with specific ingredients in specific quantities. This chapter is different.

The three master formulas here are frameworks. Each one is a core batter or dough with a set of ratios that work reliably, followed by a variation table that shows you how to change the flavor profile without changing the underlying structure. The muffin formula produces six distinct muffins from one base. The cracker formula produces six distinct crackers from one base. The pancake formula produces five distinct pancake variations from one base.

That is seventeen recipe outcomes from three master formulas. Which means by the end of this chapter, you have the equivalent of nearly sixty recipes across the whole book.

But the more important thing this chapter teaches is not the variations. It is the underlying logic: what can change in a batter without affecting the structure, and what cannot. Flour ratios, fat ratios, and leavening ratios are structural. Flavorings, mix-ins, and toppings are flexible. Once you understand which is which, you can adapt any recipe you encounter, and eventually create your own.

> *A recipe tells you what to make. A formula teaches you how baking works. This chapter is the transition between the two.*

Each master formula below includes the base recipe with full instructions, followed by a variation table. The variation table specifies only what changes from the base. Everything else stays the same.

THE MASTER MUFFIN FORMULA

This formula produces a muffin that is tender without being cakey, moist without being gummy, and structured enough to hold mix-ins without them sinking to the bottom. It is calibrated for 100% hydration discard and standard all-purpose flour. The six variations in the table below cover sweet, savory, fruit, vegetable, and indulgent directions.

INGREDIENTS - BASE FORMULA (MAKES 12 MUFFINS)

Dry Ingredients
2 cups (240 g) all-purpose flour
1/2 cup (100 g) granulated sugar
2 teaspoons (9 g) baking powder
1/2 teaspoon (3 g) baking soda
1/2 teaspoon (3 g) fine salt
Wet Ingredients
3/4 cup (180 g) sourdough discard, cold
2 large eggs
1/3 cup (80 ml) whole milk
1/3 cup (75 ml) neutral oil or melted butter
1 teaspoon (5 ml) pure vanilla extract
Mix-ins
1 1/2 cups of your chosen additions (see variation table)

INSTRUCTIONS

Base Method

1. Preheat oven to 375 degrees F (190 degrees C). Line a 12-cup muffin tin with paper liners.
2. Whisk all dry ingredients together in a large bowl until fully combined.
3. In a separate bowl, whisk all wet ingredients together until smooth.
4. Pour the wet ingredients into the dry. Fold with a spatula, counting strokes: stop at 12 to 15 strokes. The batter must be lumpy. Overmixed muffin batter develops gluten tunnels and peaked, tough tops.
5. Fold in mix-ins with 2 to 3 additional strokes.

6. Fill each muffin cup three-quarters full. Bake 20 to 22 minutes until a toothpick inserted in the center comes out with a few moist crumbs.
7. Cool in the tin 5 minutes, then transfer to a wire rack.

BAKER'S TIP

The ratio that makes this formula work is 2 cups flour to 3/4 cup discard to 2 eggs. This produces the right gluten structure for a tender muffin that holds its shape. Do not reduce the eggs or increase the discard significantly without adjusting the flour to compensate, or the muffins will be gummy in the center.

Variation Table

Use the base formula exactly as written. Apply only the changes listed below for each variation.

Variation	Swap in Dry	Swap in Wet	Mix-ins
Lemon Poppy	**Add** 1 tsp lemon zest to dry	**Replace** 2 tbsp milk with lemon juice	2 tbsp poppy seeds
Apple Cinnamon	**Add** 1 tsp cinnamon, pinch nutmeg	No change	1 cup peeled diced apple, 1/2 cup chopped walnuts
Double Chocolate	**Replace** 1/4 cup flour with cocoa powder	No change	1 cup chocolate chips
Carrot Spice	**Add** 1 tsp cinnamon, 1/4 tsp ginger, 1/4 tsp cloves	Replace oil with melted butter	1 cup grated carrot, 1/2 cup raisins
Savory Herb	**Reduce sugar to** 1 tbsp, add 1 tsp dried thyme	No change	3/4 cup feta, 1/4 cup sun-dried tomatoes (drained and chopped)

Variation	Swap in Dry	Swap in Wet	Mix-ins
Brown Butter Peach	**Add** 1/2 tsp cinnamon	Brown the oil's worth of butter (see Recipe 26); use cooled	1 cup fresh or frozen peach chunks (do not thaw if frozen)

Storage: All variations: airtight container at room temperature up to 3 days, refrigerator up to 5 days, freezer up to 3 months.

THE MASTER CRACKER FORMULA

The cracker formula is the most flexible in the chapter. Crackers are more forgiving than muffins because the structure is simpler: flour provides body, fat provides tenderness and crunch, discard provides flavor and acidity, and salt provides seasoning. Almost everything else is negotiable. The six variations below range from wholesome to indulgent to boldly spiced.

Base Formula (makes about 60 thin crackers)

INGREDIENTS

1 cup (240 g) sourdough discard, cold
1 cup (120 g) all-purpose flour (see variation table for substitutions)
3 tablespoons (42 g) unsalted butter, melted, or 3 tablespoons (45 ml) olive oil
1/2 teaspoon (3 g) fine salt
Flaky salt for topping
1 tablespoon water if needed to bring dough together

INSTRUCTIONS

Base Method

1. Preheat oven to 325 degrees F (165 degrees C).
2. Combine the discard, flour, fat, and salt. Mix until a smooth, cohesive dough forms. If crumbly, add water one teaspoon at a time.

3. Divide in half. Roll each half between two sheets of parchment to 1 to 2 mm thickness (credit card thin).
4. Slide parchment onto a baking sheet, peel off the top sheet, and score into shapes. Add toppings and press in gently.
5. Bake 18 to 22 minutes at 325 degrees F, rotating halfway, until uniformly golden and dry to the touch.
6. Cool completely on the pan before breaking apart. Crackers crisp as they cool.

BAKER'S TIP

The ratio that makes this formula work is 1:1 discard to flour by volume, with fat at roughly 15 percent of the total weight. Within those proportions, the flavor variables are almost unlimited. Change the flour type, the fat type, or the seasoning and you have a completely different cracker.

Variation Table

Use the base formula exactly as written. Apply only the changes listed for each variation.

Variation	Flour Change	Fat Change	Seasoning and Topping
Whole Wheat Sesame	**Replace** 1/2 cup AP flour with whole wheat	Use olive oil instead of butter	2 tbsp sesame seeds in dough; flaky salt on top
Black Pepper Cheddar	No change	Use butter	1 tsp coarsely ground black pepper in dough, 1/4 cup finely grated cheddar pressed into surface
Za'atar and Olive Oil	No change	Use olive oil; increase to 4 tbsp	2 tbsp za'atar spice blend mixed into dough; flaky salt on top
Rye and Caraway	**Replace** 1/3 cup AP flour with dark rye flour	Use butter	1 tsp caraway seeds in dough; flaky salt on top

Variation	Flour Change	Fat Change	Seasoning and Topping
Sweet Cinnamon	No change	Use butter	**Add** 2 tbsp sugar and 1 tsp cinnamon to dough; sprinkle turbinado sugar on top
Turmeric and Cumin	No change	Use olive oil	1/2 tsp turmeric, 1/2 tsp cumin, pinch cayenne in dough; flaky salt on top

Storage: All variations: airtight container at room temperature up to 1 week. If they soften, return to a 300 degree F oven for 5 to 8 minutes and cool completely.

THE MASTER PANCAKE FORMULA

The pancake formula is the one you should understand most deeply, because pancake batter is the entry point for the widest range of discard cooking. The structural ratio here is discard to flour to egg to liquid. Change the liquid ratio and you change the thickness. Change the flour type and you change the texture and flavor. The leavening stays fixed because it is doing precise chemical work that the other variables cannot replace.

Base Formula (makes 10 to 12 pancakes)

INGREDIENTS

1 cup (240 g) sourdough discard, cold
1 cup (120 g) all-purpose flour
1 tablespoon (12 g) granulated sugar
1 teaspoon (5 g) baking powder
1/2 teaspoon (3 g) baking soda
1/2 teaspoon (3 g) fine salt
1 large egg
3/4 cup (180 ml) whole milk
2 tablespoons (28 g) unsalted butter, melted
1 teaspoon (5 ml) pure vanilla extract

INSTRUCTIONS

Base Method

1. Whisk all dry ingredients together in a large bowl.
2. In a separate bowl, whisk all wet ingredients, including the discard, until smooth.
3. Pour wet into dry and fold until just combined. Stop as soon as the dry flour disappears. Rest 5 minutes.
4. Cook in a buttered skillet over medium heat, using 1/4 cup batter per pancake, until bubbles form across the surface and edges look set. Flip once and cook 1 to 2 more minutes.
5. Understanding the Thickness Variable
6. This formula as written produces a standard-thickness pancake: about 1 centimeter tall when fully cooked. To adjust thickness without changing the yield or flavor significantly:
7. Thicker pancakes: reduce the milk by 2 tablespoons. The batter will be stiffer and cook more slowly. Use medium-low heat and allow 3 to 4 minutes per side.
8. Thinner pancakes (closer to crepes): increase the milk by 2 to 3 tablespoons. The batter pours more easily and cooks faster. Use medium-high heat and flip after about 90 seconds.
9. Understanding the Leavening Variable
10. The combination of baking powder and baking soda is not interchangeable. Baking powder provides initial lift when mixed with liquid and again when it hits heat. Baking soda requires an acid to activate, which is why it works here: the sourdough discard provides that acid. Together they produce a pancake that rises in the pan and stays fluffy rather than deflating as it cools. Changing one without adjusting the other will affect the rise and texture significantly.

BAKER'S TIP

You can make the batter up to 12 hours ahead and refrigerate it covered. The discard continues to ferment gently in the refrigerator, which deepens the flavor. The baking soda and baking powder will also continue to react slowly, so the batter will be slightly less vigorous by morning. Add 1/4 teaspoon of fresh baking powder to the cold batter and stir gently before cooking to restore some lift.

Variation Table

Use the base formula exactly as written. Apply only the changes listed for each variation.

Variation	Thickness Adjustment	Flavor Addition	Mix-in or Topping
Buckwheat	**Replace** 1/3 cup AP flour with buckwheat flour; batter will be slightly thicker	**Add** 1 tsp honey to wet ingredients	Serve with whipped butter and maple syrup
Cardamom Orange	No change	**Add** 1/2 tsp cardamom and zest of 1 orange to batter	Top with fresh orange segments and a drizzle of honey
Peanut Butter	**Thin the batter with** 2 tbsp extra milk; peanut butter thickens it	**Whisk** 3 tbsp smooth peanut butter into wet ingredients until fully incorporated	**Fold in** 1/2 cup chocolate chips; top with sliced banana
Corn and Honey	**Replace** 1/4 cup AP flour with fine cornmeal; batter will be slightly grainier	**Add** 2 tbsp honey to wet ingredients; reduce sugar to 1/2 tbsp	Top with whipped butter and additional honey
Savory Herb Thin	**Add** 2 tbsp extra milk for a thinner, crepe-like result	Omit sugar and vanilla; add 1/2 tsp black pepper, 1 tbsp fresh thyme leaves	Serve topped with a fried egg, sliced avocado, and flaky salt

Storage: Cooked pancakes: refrigerate up to 3 days, freeze up to 2 months. Reheat in a toaster or 325 degree F oven. Uncooked batter: refrigerate up to 12 hours.

WHAT THE FORMULAS HAVE IN COMMON

Looking across all three master formulas, a pattern emerges. Each one has a fixed structural core and a flexible exterior. The muffin formula's core is the flour-to-discard-to-egg ratio. The cracker formula's core is the discard-to-flour-to-fat ratio. The pancake formula's core is the discard-to-flour-to-egg-to-liquid ratio combined with a precise leavening balance.

Everything outside those ratios is flavor. Flavorings, mix-ins, toppings, flour swaps within reasonable ranges, fat type switches, herb and spice additions: all of these change the character of the finished product without destabilizing the structure.

This is how professional bakers think, and it is a useful way to approach all of the recipes in this book. When something does not turn out as expected, the question to ask is not 'what went wrong with the recipe?' but 'which variable changed?' Most of the time the answer is in Chapter 8.

CHAPTER 8

Troubleshooting Master Guide

Every baker has a bad bake. An afternoon where the pancakes came out flat, the crackers went soft, the cake sank in the center, or the biscuits refused to rise. It happens to experienced bakers and beginners equally, and it happens for specific, identifiable reasons.

This chapter is organized by symptom, not by recipe. When something goes wrong, you are not thinking about which recipe caused the problem. You are thinking about what the problem looks like. Find your symptom in the section headings below, read the diagnosis, and apply the fix. Most issues have a cause that can be identified in about thirty seconds and a fix that takes thirty seconds more.

The chapter is divided into five sections: texture problems, flavor problems, baking and oven problems, discard problems, and scaling and substitution problems. Each section addresses the most common failures in that category with three pieces of information: the cause (what actually went wrong, mechanically), the fix (what to do right now or next time), and the prevention (how to stop it from happening again).

> *A recipe that fails once and teaches you something is more valuable than ten recipes that succeed without explanation. Use this chapter. It is the part of the book that makes everything else more reliable.*

A note before you begin: many baking problems have more than one possible cause. If the first cause listed does not match your situation, read through to the second and third. The most common cause is listed first, but baking is a system, and systems can fail at multiple points simultaneously.

SECTION 1: TEXTURE PROBLEMS

> *Texture problems are the most common category of baking failure and also the most diagnosable. The texture of a baked good is a direct record of what happened during mixing, resting, and baking. Once you know what to look for, the baked good itself tells you what went wrong.*

The baked good is too dense or gummy in the center

Cause:
Most likely: undermixing of wet and dry ingredients left pockets of unhydrated flour, which cooked into dense patches. Second possibility: the recipe was underbaked. Third possibility: too much discard relative to flour unbalanced the wet-to-dry ratio.

Fix:
If the center is gummy and the edges are cooked: return to the oven at the same temperature, loosely tented with foil to prevent over-browning, for 8 to 12 additional minutes. Test again with a toothpick. If the whole thing is dense rather than just gummy in spots: the issue is mixing or ratio, not baking time.

Prevention:
For muffins and quick breads, mix wet and dry together until just combined and no dry streaks remain. Gummy spots are almost always unhydrated flour. For pancakes, let the batter rest 5 minutes after mixing so the flour fully hydrates before cooking.

✦ ✦ ✦

The baked good is too dry or crumbly

Cause:
Too much flour relative to liquid, or overbaking, or both. In cracker and shortbread recipes, it can also mean the fat was too cold and did not distribute evenly through the dough.

Fix:
There is no fix for an already dry baked good, but you can repurpose it: dry muffins crumbled into yogurt or ice cream are good. Dry cake layers work in a trifle with plenty of cream or custard. For next time: measure flour by spooning it into the measuring cup and leveling off, rather than scooping the cup directly into the flour bag, which compacts it and adds 10 to 20 percent more flour than the recipe intends.

Prevention:
Use a scale. Weight is the only reliable measurement for flour. Alternatively, use the spoon-and-level method for cups. Do not scoop directly from the bag.

✦ ✦ ✦

Muffins have large tunnels or peaked, tough tops

Cause:
Overmixing. When muffin batter is mixed beyond the point where the flour disappears, gluten strands develop and become elastic. Gas produced by the leavening cannot escape through the elastic batter evenly, so it shoots upward through the path of least resistance, creating tall peaked tops and long vertical tunnels inside.

Fix:
There is no fix for this in the current batch. The structure is set. Next time: count your strokes. Twelve to fifteen folds maximum after the wet ingredients go into the dry. Stop when you can no longer see dry flour. Lumps are fine. Lumps are correct.

Prevention:
Use a spatula rather than a whisk for muffin batter. A whisk incorporates air

✦ ✦ ✦

Cookies spread too much and are thin and crispy when you wanted thick and chewy

Cause:

The butter was too warm (or melted), which means it spread in the oven before the structure could set. Second possibility: too much sugar relative to flour. Third: the baking sheet was warm from a previous batch.

Fix:

Refrigerate the remaining dough for 30 minutes before baking the next batch. Use a cold baking sheet. If the butter was melted or very soft, the spread cookies are likely still edible but will not have the intended texture.

Prevention:

Chill cookie dough before baking whenever the recipe calls for it. Use room-temperature butter for creamed cookie doughs, not softened-past-the-point-of-squishy butter. Always start with a cold baking sheet.

✦ ✦ ✦

Cookies do not spread enough and are thick, dry pucks

Cause:

The butter was too cold, or too much flour was added, or the dough was over-chilled before baking.

Fix:

Press the balls of dough down lightly with the palm of your hand before baking to encourage spread. For the next batch, let the dough warm for 10 minutes before scooping.

Prevention:

For creamed cookie doughs, use butter at true room temperature: it should leave an indentation when pressed with a finger but not squish immediately. Cold butter does not cream properly with sugar and produces a stiff dough that resists spread.

✦ ✦ ✦

Crackers are chewy or soft after cooling instead of crispy

Cause:

Most likely: underbaked. Crackers need to be fully dry throughout, not just golden on the outside. Second: stored in an airtight container while still slightly warm, which traps steam and softens them. Third: stored in the refrigerator, where humidity softens them overnight.

Fix:

Return soft crackers to a 300 degree F oven for 8 to 10 minutes. Let cool completely on the pan, uncovered, before storing. They will re-crisp fully.

Prevention:

Do not judge cracker doneness by color alone. They should feel dry and rigid when you press the center gently. Let them cool completely, at least 20 minutes, before moving to an airtight container. Never refrigerate crackers.

✦ ✦ ✦

Bread or flatbread is tough and chewy rather than tenderCause: Overworked dough. In recipes that call for minimal mixing or no kneading, additional working after the dough comes together develops gluten that makes the finished product dense and tough. This is especially common in biscuits, scones, flatbreads, and pizza doughs.

Fix:
There is no fix for overworked dough once it is baked. For next time: in recipes that specify minimal mixing, take that instruction literally. The dough should just barely hold together. Rough and shaggy is correct for biscuits and scones. Smooth and polished means you went too far.

Prevention:
Use a light touch and count your mixing actions. Biscuit dough: press and fold, not knead. Flatbread dough: minimal kneading, a few minutes at most. The goal is incorporation, not development.

SECTION 2: FLAVOR PROBLEMS

> *Flavor problems in sourdough discard baking almost always trace back to one variable: the discard itself. Its age, sourness, and hydration level affect every recipe it enters. The good news is that once you identify the flavor problem, the source is usually obvious and the fix for next time is simple.*

Everything tastes too sour

Cause:
The discard was too old or too tangy for the recipe. Assertive discard (7 or more days old) has enough acidity to overpower delicate recipes. The sourness in discard increases linearly with time in the refrigerator and accelerates in warm conditions.

Fix: For the current batch: add a small amount of extra sugar or fat, both of which suppress the perception of acidity. An extra tablespoon of butter folded into pancake batter, or an additional tablespoon of sugar in a muffin, can noticeably soften aggressive sourness. For next time: use younger discard in delicate recipes.

Prevention:
Run the Quick Discard Assessment from Chapter 2 before every bake. Match the sourness profile of your discard to the recipe category. Tangy discard belongs in crackers, flatbreads, and chocolate cake. It does not belong in shortbread, crepes, or delicate muffins.

✦ ✦ ✦

The baked good tastes flat or bland despite following the recipe

Cause:
Most likely: underseasoning. Salt is the primary flavor enhancer in baking and the most commonly under-measured ingredient. Second possibility: the discard was very mild and contributed less flavor than expected. Third: vanilla extract was old or low quality.

Fix:
For a baked good that is already made: there is limited recovery, but a sprinkle of flaky salt on top of a muffin, pancake, or cracker can do more than you expect. For the batter or dough itself: taste it before baking. Raw batter and dough should taste slightly over-salted, because baking mellows salt perception.

Prevention:
Measure salt accurately. Use a scale for small amounts. Use a mid-aged discard (4 to 7 days) for maximum flavor contribution. Replace vanilla extract if it has been open for more than 2 years.

✦ ✦ ✦

There is an off or unpleasant flavor that is not simply sournessCause:The discard itself. An off flavor in the finished bake almost always originates in the discard. Possible causes: discard that has gone slightly bad without visible signs, discard stored in a container that retained odors from previous contents, or discard from a starter that was fed with rancid flour.

Fix:
Taste the discard before adding it to any recipe. Discard should taste tangy, slightly sour, and complex. Any chemical, rancid, medicinal, or genuinely unpleasant flavor in the discard will appear in the baked good and there is no way to correct it after the fact.

Prevention:
Always smell and taste your discard before baking. Store discard in clean, odor-free jars. Feed your starter with fresh flour from a sealed container. When in doubt about discard quality, start fresh.

✦ ✦ ✦

Sweet recipes taste inexplicably wrong, almost metallic or bitter

Cause:
Too much baking soda. Baking soda requires acid to neutralize it. In discard recipes, the discard provides some of that acid, but if the recipe calls for more baking soda than the discard can neutralize, the excess soda remains active and produces a soapy, bitter, or metallic aftertaste. This is more common with very mild discard that has less acidity than expected.

Fix:
For the current batch: there is no fix. For next time, if your discard is consistently mild: reduce baking soda by 1/8 teaspoon and add 1/4 teaspoon of baking powder as a replacement. Baking powder contains its own acid and does not need the discard's acidity to activate.

Prevention:

Measure baking soda precisely. The difference between 1/2 teaspoon and 1 teaspoon of baking soda is significant. Use a measuring spoon and level it off. More is not better.

SECTION 3: BAKING AND OVEN PROBLEMS

> *Oven problems are frequently misdiagnosed as recipe problems. Before concluding that a recipe does not work, consider whether the oven itself is the variable. Most home ovens run 25 to 50 degrees hotter or cooler than the set temperature, and many cycle significantly around their target temperature. An inexpensive oven thermometer costs under ten dollars and resolves more baking problems than any other single tool.*

The outside burns before the inside is cooked through

Cause:

The oven is running hot, the pan is too dark (dark pans absorb more heat), or the bake is placed too close to the heat source. For cakes and quick breads specifically, this can also mean the batter was too cold when it went into the oven.

Fix:

Tent the bake loosely with aluminum foil to shield the exterior from direct heat and continue baking until the interior is cooked through. For next time: use an oven thermometer to verify your actual oven temperature and adjust accordingly.

Prevention:

Buy an oven thermometer. Set your oven 25 degrees lower if you notice consistent burning on the exterior before the interior is done. Use light-colored aluminum pans rather than dark nonstick pans for cakes and muffins. Place pans in the center of the oven, not on the highest rack.

✦ ✦ ✦

The bake is pale and underdone even at the specified time

Cause:

The oven is running cool. This is as common as running hot and produces the opposite problem: extended bake times produce dried-out exteriors by the time the interior is finally cooked through. Second possibility: the pan is too thick and insulating, preventing heat from reaching the batter.

Fix:

Increase the oven temperature by 25 degrees and continue baking. Check every 5 minutes. Use an oven thermometer to establish a baseline for your oven's actual temperature.

Prevention:

Calibrate your oven. Place an oven thermometer in the center of the oven at your typical baking temperature and leave it for 20 minutes. Note the actual temperature. Adjust your settings for every recipe accordingly.

✦ ✦ ✦

Baked goods are cooked unevenly, with one side darker than the other

Cause:

Hot spots in the oven. Every oven has them, particularly near the back wall and near the heating element. Oven hot spots are normal and expected.

Fix:

Rotate baking pans 180 degrees halfway through the baking time. This is mentioned in several recipes in this book and should be a default habit for anything baked at high heat for more than 15 minutes.

Prevention:Rotate everything, always. Place pans in the center of the oven rather than close to any wall. If one oven rack position consistently produces better results than another, note it and use it by default.

Crackers burn at the edges before the center crisps

Cause:

The crackers are not rolled to an even thickness. Thinner areas cook faster and burn before thicker areas are done. This is the most common cracker problem and has nothing to do with the recipe or the oven temperature.

Fix:

Remove the crackers from the edges of the pan that are burning, and return the center pieces for additional time. For next time: roll more carefully, checking thickness by holding the rolled dough up to light. You will see the thicker and thinner areas clearly.

Prevention:

Roll cracker dough between two sheets of parchment, rotating the dough 90 degrees every few passes, to distribute any uneven pressure. Work from the center outward. Check the edges last, as they tend to thin out when rolling.

Cake or quick bread sinks in the center after baking

Cause:

Most likely: underbaked. The center was not set when removed from the oven, and it collapsed as it cooled. Second: too much leavening, which creates a rapid initial rise that the structure cannot support. Third: the oven door was opened during the first half of baking, causing a temperature drop that deflated the rise.

Fix:
A sunken cake is structurally fine to eat. Fill the depression with frosting, whipped cream, or fruit. For next time: test doneness with a toothpick inserted in the actual center, not near the edge. The center takes longer to set than the edges.

Prevention:
Do not open the oven door during the first two-thirds of baking time. Set a timer for the minimum bake time and resist checking before it goes off. Measure leavening precisely.

✦ ✦ ✦

SECTION 4: DISCARD PROBLEMS

> *Problems with the discard itself are the most upstream failure point in this book's recipes. Everything else can be adjusted. But if the discard is wrong, fixing the downstream recipe is working in the wrong direction. Always start with the discard assessment from Chapter 2.*

The discard has a thick grey or brown liquid layer on top

Cause:
This is hooch, a completely normal byproduct of fermentation. Yeast produces alcohol as a byproduct of eating flour, and that alcohol collects on top of the denser discard. It is not a sign of spoilage. It is a sign of a healthy, active, older discard.

Fix:
Stir it back in. The hooch adds a slight flavor complexity and no harm whatsoever. If you prefer, pour it off before using the discard, but this is purely a preference decision.

Prevention:
Hooch forms naturally in any discard that sits for more than a few days. There is nothing to prevent. It is not a problem.

✦ ✦ ✦

The discard has separated into a solid layer and a watery liquid that will not stir back together

Cause:

The discard has been frozen and thawed, or has been in the refrigerator for a very long time (more than 2 weeks). The protein structure has broken down enough that it no longer holds as an emulsion. This is different from hooch.

Fix:

Stir vigorously. If it re-emulsifies, use it in strongly flavored recipes like crackers or chocolate cake where any textural oddity will not be noticeable. If it does not come back together after extended stirring, it is past its useful life.

Prevention:

Use discard within 2 weeks of refrigeration or freeze promptly after the first week. Label frozen discard with the date.

✦ ✦ ✦

The discard smells wrong: not just sour, but genuinely unpleasant

Cause:

The discard has spoiled. This can happen if the starter itself was contaminated, if the jar was not clean, if the discard was left at room temperature too long, or if it has been in the refrigerator for more than 3 weeks. Pink, orange, red, or black streaks or patches are a definitive sign of contamination.

Fix:

Throw it away. Do not taste it to confirm. An unpleasant smell is sufficient reason to discard. Clean the jar thoroughly with hot water and soap before starting fresh.

Prevention:

Use clean jars. Smell and taste discard before every use. Refrigerate within a few hours of feeding. Use within 2 weeks or freeze.

✦ ✦ ✦

The discard is much thicker than expected, almost like bread dough

Cause:

Your starter is maintained at a lower hydration than 100 percent, meaning more flour relative to water is used at each feeding. This is common with stiff starters, which some bakers prefer for other reasons.

Fix:

Thin the discard with water before measuring. Add water a tablespoon at a time, stirring between additions, until it reaches a pourable, thick-batter consistency. Then measure the amount the recipe calls for. This produces the equivalent of 100 percent hydration discard for recipe purposes.

Prevention:

Note your starter's hydration and apply this adjustment automatically every time you use it in this book's recipes. It is a quick step that makes every recipe more predictable.

✦ ✦ ✦

You ran out of discard halfway through a recipe

Cause:

The recipe needed more than you had available.

Fix:For most recipes in this book, you can substitute plain yogurt, buttermilk, or a mixture of equal parts plain yogurt and water for the missing portion of discard. These substitutes provide similar acidity and liquid content. The flavor will be slightly less complex but the texture will be correct.

Prevention:
Check discard quantity before starting any recipe. If you are close to the minimum amount needed, add a teaspoon of apple cider vinegar to yogurt or milk as a rough substitute for any shortfall. Freeze discard in measured portions so you always know exactly how much you have available.

SECTION 5: SCALING AND SUBSTITUTION

> *Scaling recipes and substituting ingredients are the two most common sources of baking problems among home bakers who are comfortable with recipes but not yet comfortable with the underlying principles. This section addresses the most frequent scaling and substitution questions across the recipes in this book.*

I halved the recipe but the bake time seems wrong

Cause:
Halving a recipe changes the volume of batter but not the thickness of what you put in the pan. If you use a smaller pan to compensate, the depth of the batter stays similar and bake times are approximately the same. If you use the same pan, the batter is shallower and will cook faster.

Fix:
When halving a recipe, use a pan that is proportionally smaller to maintain approximately the same batter depth. For cakes, a round 6-inch pan instead of a 9-inch pan. For muffins, fill 6 cups of the tin instead of 12. Begin checking for doneness 5 minutes earlier than the recipe specifies.

Prevention: Think of bake time as determined primarily by the depth of the batter, not the total volume. Same depth means approximately same time. Shallower means faster.

✦ ✦ ✦

I doubled the recipe and it did not turn out as well as the single batch

Cause:

Two possible issues. First: doubled batter in the same pan is too deep and the heat cannot penetrate to the center in the standard bake time. Second: doubled leavening sometimes slightly over-leavens, producing a rapid rise that collapses. Third: mixing a larger volume in the same bowl means more likelihood of incomplete incorporation.

Fix:

For doubled cake or quick bread recipes: use two pans rather than one larger pan and bake simultaneously. For doubled cookie or cracker doughs: chill between batches if the dough becomes warm from extended handling.

Prevention:

When doubling, maintain the same pan dimensions and use more pans rather than deeper pans. Leavening scales almost linearly, but if you notice excessive rise and collapse when doubling, reduce the total leavening by 10 percent.

✦ ✦ ✦

I substituted whole wheat flour for all-purpose and the result was dense and heavy

Cause:

Whole wheat flour contains bran, which cuts through gluten strands during mixing. This limits gluten development and produces a denser crumb than all-purpose flour alone. Whole wheat also absorbs more liquid, which further densifies the result.

Fix:
In future attempts: substitute a maximum of one-third of the all-purpose flour with whole wheat, not all of it. Increase liquid by one tablespoon per quarter cup of whole wheat flour added. If you want a fully whole wheat recipe, look specifically for whole wheat recipes that have been calibrated for it.

Prevention:
Use whole wheat flour as a partial replacement rather than a full substitution. The one-third whole wheat to two-thirds all-purpose ratio produces a noticeably heartier result with improved flavor without the density of a full whole wheat substitution.

✦ ✦ ✦

I substituted a gluten-free flour blend and the texture is wrong

Cause:
Gluten-free flour blends vary enormously in composition and absorptive capacity. Many contain xanthan gum, rice flour, and potato starch in varying ratios. A 1:1 substitution rarely works because gluten-free flours behave very differently from all-purpose flour in hydration, binding, and structure.

Fix:
Gluten-free baking is a different discipline from standard baking and requires recipes written specifically for gluten free flours. The recipes in this book are not gluten-free recipes and are not designed to accommodate 1:1 gluten-free substitutions. Several recipes in this book are naturally lower in gluten (the Socca flatbread in Chapter 4, for example), and these are better starting points for gluten-sensitive bakers.

Prevention:
Use recipes designed for gluten-free flours rather than substituting in standard recipes. The chemistry is genuinely different and the results of direct substitution are unpredictable.

✦ ✦ ✦

I want to make a recipe dairy-free. What can I substitute?

Cause:

Not a problem, a question. Dairy substitutions work well in most of this book's recipes, with some variation in texture and flavor.

Fix:

For milk: use oat milk or full-fat coconut milk in a 1:1 ratio. Almond milk and rice milk are too thin and watery for most recipes. For butter: use refined coconut oil in a 1:1 ratio by weight for most applications. Vegan butter sticks also work well. For cream: full-fat coconut cream is the most reliable substitute for heavy cream in batters and frostings. For cream cheese (in the cinnamon roll glaze): vegan cream cheese works in a 1:1 ratio.

Prevention:

No prevention needed. Dairy-free substitutions are built into the recipe adjustments above. The flavor will be slightly different in some recipes, particularly those where butter is a primary flavor contributor (shortbread, brown butter cake), but the texture will be correct.

USING THIS CHAPTER PROACTIVELY

Most bakers use a troubleshooting guide reactively: something went wrong, so they look it up. That is exactly the right use of this chapter. But there is a more powerful approach.

Read through the sections that cover the recipe types you make most often before you make them. The texture section before your first batch of muffins. The cracker section before your first crackers. The discard section before you use discard that has been sitting for more than a week. Ten minutes of reading now prevents an hour of frustration later.

The causes listed in this chapter are not guesses. They are the actual mechanical explanations for the failures described. If you understand why something happens rather than just what to do about it, you will be able to diagnose problems this guide does not specifically address, because you will understand the system well enough to identify where it broke down.

That is the goal. Not to turn you into someone who never has a bad bake. Bad bakes will always happen. The goal is to turn you into someone who knows exactly why a bad bake happened and how to prevent it next time. Which is, after all, how every good baker got good.

CHAPTER 9

Reference Materials

The five reference tables in this section are designed to be used repeatedly rather than read once. Bookmark this section or fold down the corner of the page. The discard index and occasion index in particular will answer the question most bakers face at least once a week: what should I make with what I have?

APPENDIX A: DISCARD STORAGE REFERENCE

A quick reference for how to store discard, how long each method lasts, and what warning signs indicate discard that should not be used. For the full assessment system, see Chapter 2.

Method	Container	Lifespan	Warning Signs	Before Using	Best Recipes
Refrigerator	Glass jar with loose lid	**Up to** 2 weeks	Pink or black spots; foul smell	Stir in hooch; run Chapter 2 assessment	Any recipe
Freezer	Zip-lock bag or glass jar with headspace	**Up to** 3 months	Separation that won't re-emulsify after thawing	Thaw overnight in refrigerator; stir well	Crackers, flatbreads, muffins
Room temperature	Glass jar, loosely covered	12 to 24 hours max	Rapid hooch buildup; strong alcohol smell after several hours	Use immediately; more active than refrigerator discard	Pancakes, waffles, flatbreads

Method	Container	Lifespan	Warning Signs	Before Using	Best Recipes
Frozen portions	Ice cube trays, then transfer to bags	**Up to** 3 months	Same as freezer above	Thaw quantity needed; combine cubes	Efficient for small-batch recipes

A note on the refrigerator lifespan: two weeks is the conservative, reliable limit. Many experienced bakers use refrigerator discard up to three weeks old with good results, particularly in strongly flavored recipes like crackers or chocolate cake. Trust your nose and the Chapter 2 smell test over any arbitrary date limit.

✦ ✦ ✦

APPENDIX B: DISCARD SUBSTITUTION GUIDE

For times when you are out of discard, or need to use a substitute for a portion of the discard a recipe calls for. These substitutes replicate the acidity and approximate liquid content of discard. They cannot replicate its flavor complexity, but they will produce structurally correct results.

If you need	Best substitute	Ratio	Notes
1 cup discard	1/2 cup plain yogurt + 1/2 cup all-purpose flour	1:1 total volume	Closest in acidity and texture. Use full-fat yogurt for best results.
1 cup discard	1/2 cup buttermilk + 1/2 cup all-purpose flour	1:1 total volume	Works well in pancakes, muffins, and quick breads. Slightly less tangy than discard.
1 cup discard (in crackers only)	1/2 cup sour cream + 1/4 cup water + 1/4 cup flour	1:1 total volume	Higher fat content changes cracker texture slightly; produces a more tender cracker.

If you need	Best substitute	Ratio	Notes
The sourness of discard only	**Add** 1 tsp apple cider vinegar per 1/4 cup of plain milk or water	1 tsp vinegar per 1/4 cup liquid	Activates baking soda and adds acidity without the discard's flavor complexity.
Active starter (not discard)	Discard works in most cases with adjusted leavening	1:1 plus 1/4 tsp extra baking powder	Discard has less active yeast than a fed starter. Add baking powder to compensate in non-yeasted recipes.

The yogurt plus flour combination is the closest substitute to discard in terms of behavior across all recipe categories. It is worth keeping plain full-fat yogurt in the refrigerator as a backup whenever your discard supply is unreliable.

APPENDIX C: RECIPE INDEX BY OCCASION

The occasion index answers the question you actually have, which is rarely about discard age and more often about what you are making and why. Use this alongside Appendix C: find your occasion, then cross-reference the discard profile your current discard falls into.

Occasion	Recipes
Weekday breakfast (under 30 min)	01 Classic Pancakes, 03 Savory Scallion Pancakes, 04 Belgian Waffles, 11 Crepes, 12 Hash Browns, 13 Breakfast Fritters
Weekend brunch	02 Blueberry Lemon Ricotta Pancakes, 05 Overnight Oat Waffles, 14 Sourdough Biscuits, 32 Cinnamon Rolls, 33 Crepe Cake
Snacks and grazing boards	15 through 20 (all crackers), 40 Breadsticks, 39 Soft Pretzels, 17 Parmesan Rosemary Crackers, 19 Sesame Miso Crackers
Weeknight dinner sides	21 Same-Day Flatbread, 22 Pizza Dough, 23 Pita-Style Bread, 24 Socca, 41 Ham and Gruyere Scones, 42 Sheet Pan Focaccia

Occasion	Recipes
Entertaining and special occasions	25 Sourdough Chocolate Cake, 26 Brown Butter Banana Cake, 27 Olive Oil Citrus Cake, 32 Cinnamon Rolls, 33 Crepe Cake, 34 Tart Shell, 39 Soft Pretzels
Gifts and bake sales	15 through 20 (all crackers), 28 Chocolate Chip Cookies, 29 Snickerdoodles, 30 Brownies, 31 Shortbread, 06 Master Muffins (any variation)
No-bake or minimal effort	33 No-Bake Crepe Cake (assembly only), 01 Classic Pancakes, 11 Crepes, 21 Same-Day Flatbread, 13 Breakfast Fritters
Using up large amounts of discard quickly	42 Sheet Pan Focaccia (uses 1/2 cup), 15 Master Cracker doubled (uses 2 cups), 06 Master Muffin doubled (uses 1.5 cups), 03 Savory Scallion Pancakes batch

APPENDIX D: MEASUREMENT CONVERSIONS

Weight measurements produce more consistent results than volume measurements because they are unaffected by how tightly you pack a measuring cup or how humid the air is. The table below gives weight equivalents for the most common ingredients in this book. A digital kitchen scale that can switch between grams and ounces costs less than most specialty baking tools and is the single most reliable investment you can make in consistent results.

Common Ingredient Weights

Ingredient	1 cup (volume)	1/2 cup (volume)	1 tbsp (volume)
All-purpose flour	120 g	60 g	8 g
Whole wheat flour	130 g	65 g	8 g
Rye flour	102 g	51 g	6 g
Sourdough discard	240 g	120 g	15 g
Granulated sugar	200 g	100 g	12 g
Brown sugar (packed)	220 g	110 g	14 g
Powdered sugar	120 g	60 g	8 g
Cocoa powder	85 g	43 g	5 g
Unsalted butter, melted	226 g	113 g	14 g
Olive oil / neutral oil	216 g	108 g	14 g
Whole milk	240 g	120 g	15 g
Honey / maple syrup	340 g	170 g	21 g
Rolled oats	90 g	45 g	6 g
Chocolate chips	170 g	85 g	11 g

Oven Temperature Conversions

All recipes in this book give temperatures in Fahrenheit first, with Celsius in parentheses. The table below covers the full range of temperatures used across the book.

Fahrenheit	Celsius	Common Use
275 degrees F	135 degrees C	Warming / low slow bakes
300 degrees F	150 degrees C	Re-crisping crackers, low meringues
325 degrees F	165 degrees C	Crackers, shortbread, delicate cakes
350 degrees F	175 degrees C	Cakes, muffins, loaves, cookies
375 degrees F	190 degrees C	Muffins (high dome), cookies, scones
400 degrees F	205 degrees C	Biscuits, scones, pizza (thicker)
425 degrees F	220 degrees C	Focaccia, flatbreads, pretzels
450 degrees F	230 degrees C	Pizza, high-heat flatbreads, crackers (final crisp)
475 degrees F	245 degrees C	Thin crust pizza

Quick Volume Conversions

3 teaspoons = 1 tablespoon

4 tablespoons = 1/4 cup

5 tablespoons + 1 teaspoon = 1/3 cup

8 tablespoons = 1/2 cup

16 tablespoons = 1 cup

2 cups = 1 pint

4 cups = 1 quart

1 fluid ounce = 2 tablespoons = 30 ml

1 cup = 240 ml

Pan Size Equivalents

8x8-inch square pan = approximately equal to a 9-inch round pan in batter volume

9x13-inch pan = approximately equal to two 9-inch round pans

9x5-inch loaf pan = standard loaf; holds approximately 6 cups of batter

12-cup muffin tin = standard; each cup holds approximately 1/3 cup of batter when filled three-quarters full

Half sheet pan (18x13 inches) = standard rimmed baking sheet

A FINAL NOTE

The most important thing about sourdough discard is that it makes baking more sustainable, not more complicated. Every recipe in this book was chosen because it uses an ingredient that most starter-keepers already have in excess and would otherwise throw away. The fact that the results are also genuinely good is the point.

There is no ideal baker this book is written for. The person who makes pancakes every Saturday with whatever discard has accumulated that week is using this book correctly. So is the person who made the chocolate cake once for a dinner party and wants to know what to do with the leftover jar. So is the person who read Chapter 7 and is now designing their own cracker variations based on the master formula.

Keep baking. Keep the jar. The discard will be ready when you are.

ABOUT THE AUTHOR

LeeAnn Baker is a passionate advocate for personal growth and well-being. With a deep interest in holistic self-care practices, she is dedicated to helping individuals lead healthier, more balanced lives. Through her writing, LeeAnn explores practical and effective approaches to living with purpose, fostering resilience, and nurturing mental and physical health.

When she's not writing, LeeAnn enjoys spending time outdoors, practicing mindfulness, and connecting with loved ones. She believes that everyone has the power to create positive change in their lives and is committed to inspiring others to take charge of their well-being. In addition to her focus on personal care, LeeAnn has a deep love of cooking and preserving food, finding joy in creating nourishing meals and sharing them with friends and family.

Made in the USA
Monee, IL
02 November 2026

67384028R00085